1994
Happy New Year
Love, Matthew & Dad
To Grant & Annette

THE
PYRAMID
COOKBOOK

Best wishes,

Pat Baird

12·93

Also by Pat Baird

Quick Harvest:
A Vegetarian's Guide to Microwave Cooking
(1991)

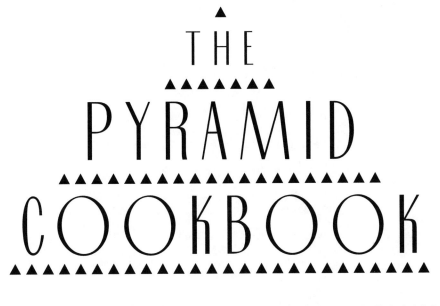

THE PYRAMID COOKBOOK

PLEASURES OF THE FOOD GUIDE PYRAMID

PAT BAIRD

HENRY HOLT AND COMPANY ▲ NEW YORK

Henry Holt and Company, Inc.
Publishers since 1866
115 West 18th Street
New York, New York 10011

Henry Holt® is a registered
trademark of Henry Holt and Company, Inc.

Published in Canada by Fitzhenry & Whiteside Ltd.,
195 Allstate Parkway, Markham, Ontario L3R 4T8.

Library of Congress Cataloging-in-Publication Data
Baird, Pat.
The pyramid cookbook: pleasures of the food guide pyramid/
Pat Baird.—1st ed.
p.   cm.
Includes bibliographical references and index.
1. Nutrition.   2. Diet.   3. Low-fat diet—Recipes.   4. High-fiber
diet—Recipes.   I. Title.
RA784.B245   1993
613.2—dc20   93-1626
                                                          CIP

ISBN 0-8050-2648-7

Henry Holt books are available for special promotions and
premiums. For details contact: Director, Special Markets.

First Edition—1993

Designed by Katy Riegel

Printed in the United States of America
All first editions are printed on acid-free paper.∞

1   3   5   7   9   10   8   6   4   2

The recipes for Linguine with Shrimp and Broccoli and Gingered Fruit Compote
were first published in *Redbook* © 1992 and are printed by permission.
The recipe for Swiss Chard Soup is adapted from
Soup, Beautiful Soup by Felipé Rojas-Lombardi
and is printed by permission of Henry Holt and Company.

To my father,
who promised me that a career
in food would always serve me well.
And it has.

▲▲▲▲▲▲▲▲▲▲▲▲▲▲▲▲▲▲▲▲▲▲▲▲▲▲▲▲▲▲▲▲▲▲▲▲▲

CONTENTS

▲▲▲

ACKNOWLEDGMENTS

Writing this book has been a real adventure for me. From the moment I heard that a new illustration was in the works to guide Americans in their food choices, I was intrigued. When the Food Guide Pyramid was introduced I knew this would be an issue that would be controversial, confusing, and challenging both to the public and to nutrition educators who would need to clarify the fine points and basic messages of the Pyramid.

Luckily, there were others who were as intrigued and excited about this as I was. I was fortunate to have lots of support, and I'd like to say thanks to everyone who helped me along the way.

Alice Martell, my agent, was ecstatic from the moment she read the proposal. She lost no time in finding a home for this book and was always responsive to any question or doubt I ever had.

Beth Crossman, my editor, wanted this book from the very first moment. Her patience, kindness, and sharp eye helped to shape and refine the manuscript into a book beyond what I had hoped it would be.

Helen Berman has unfailingly shown me the light at the end of the tunnel and gently guided me around every corner. She assisted me with this book from proposal to publication, not to mention a few other pre and post events.

Linda London (Linda London Designs, New York City) designed and reorganized my workspace in a way that truly helped me keep my sanity through this book and several other projects.

Lorna Sass after ten years continues to be a friend and colleague whose support and encouragement seem to know no limits. Her suggestions for this book always gave me a better sense of clarity and direction.

Dana Schwartz gets a special accolade for her endless phone calls, interviews, and compilation of the chapter on eating out. In addition to her duties at *Country Living* magazine and pursuit of a master's degree at New York University, she found time to give this section a national perspective to benefit readers everywhere.

Susanne Speranza is a typist, word processor, and organizer that no author should be without. She was always one step ahead of me, never let me panic (even when I wanted to), and spent many weekends and evenings getting this book the way she wanted it to be. Thanks, too, to Bob and Bobby Speranza for sharing her with me so often.

Every cookbook needs its team of tasters, and mine was a good one. Accolades to Jane Cooper, Cristina Turner, Ken Witt, Arnold Berliner, Steve Grundstein, the Bennetts, the Charwats, and the Yanis. Your comments and company are always appreciated. The constraints of opposite coasts unfortunately prevented my sister Rita from plunging her fork into each recipe, but that hardly precluded her input. She always had great comments—especially on the Asian dishes—and even tested a few recipes I faxed to her.

There are no words with which I can adequately thank everyone at USDA for the time and effort they gave me on this book. Susan Welsh, Anne Shaw, and Diane Odland were enormously helpful in the early stages. They supplied me with reports, background information, and access to whatever I needed to fully understand the Food Pyramid and its history. Even on the telephone, they spent all the time I needed to clarify certain points. Anne was thorough in reviewing the sections on servings and each of the food categories. Later, Carole Davis, Lois Fulton, Myrtle Hogbin, and Ruth Vettel went through the recipes, headnotes, and Pyramid equivalents in precise detail, giving valuable feedback. All of their efforts have truly improved the scope and accuracy of this book.

So many people in the food industry were generous with their time, products, and information. Among them are Kay Loughrey, R.D., of the National Cancer Institute, and Brian Krieg of the Produce for Better Health Foundation, who, along with Nancy Tringali, provided lots of assistance on the "5 a Day" chapter. Many others were always ready help with whatever it was I needed, including Linda Funk of the Wisconsin Milk Marketing Board; Donna Schmidt of the National Livestock and Meat Board; Bev Reyner of American Airlines; Sue Borra, R.D., of the Food Marketing Institute; Anne Salisbury, R.C., of Auletta/Perdue Farms; Denis Spanek of Spanek Inc.; Lenore Freeman of Millhopper Marketing; Norman Schoenfeld of Meyer Corporation (Slide-X cookware); Magefesa USA; Broken Arrow Ranch; The Yogurt Association; and Evans Kraft.

▲▲

THE FOOD GUIDE PYRAMID

At last, there is a new way to look at how you eat. It's the healthy way to go and, best of all, it includes all your favorite foods. It's not a gimmick and not a new diet. It is the Food Guide Pyramid, released by the United States Department of Agriculture (USDA) in 1992. It is an illustration of the USDA's Food Guide, which was developed to put the "Dietary Guidelines for Americans" into action. These guidelines are the government's official advice on how to achieve a healthy diet. (See page 2.) Finally, there is a clear *picture* of what it means to have more whole grains, breads, fruits, and vegetables, and less (not none of) fats, oils, and sugar.

The real phenomenon, though, is that the Pyramid comes at a time when Americans are giving up their notions of sacrifice and deprivation and opting for taste and pleasure. Gone is the "no pain, no gain" mentality of the eighties. Interest in health and nutrition prevails, but the mantra of the nineties is centered more around the notion of balance and moderation. Long, grueling marathons and hard-hitting, high-impact aerobics are giving way to weight training, low-impact/step aerobics, walking, swimming, and biking. Though almost everyone is concerned about fat and cholesterol in their diets, people are now willing to occasionally trade off some part of their meal for a high-fat dessert. Home cooks are trying to use woks and grills to "bring back the beef"—which they serve in smaller amounts, and then add more vegetables, breads, and grains to fill up plates. Real food with real flavor is the new food commandment. And pleasure is the motivating factor.

The experience of pleasure is an interesting part of eating. It's often said that "we eat with our eyes," and so food should first be colorful, attractive, and well presented to enhance our enjoyment. It came as something of a surprise to me, a

1

food and health professional, that appearance and taste can affect the way in which food and nutrients are absorbed. A study done by a Swedish researcher showed that iron absorption levels were higher when people ate attractively presented food than when they were given the same foods that were first puréed in a blender.

Many people want to follow the suggestions of health professionals and the advice of the Dietary Guidelines, but a lot of confusion remains about how to eat in a nutritious way and still enjoy it. In every one of my classes, workshops, or seminars, several participants bring up the notion that "if it tastes good it can't be good for you," or that deprivation and diet are the same things. People are seeking clarification as they try to refocus on the idea of what one market-research company calls "Balanced Values." This concept claims Americans are blending traditional (hard, stringent) values with newer, moderate ones where rules diminish and flexibility moves in.

▲▲

DIETARY GUIDELINES FOR AMERICANS

There are seven guidelines for a healthful diet for healthy Americans two years of age and older. They were developed jointly by USDA and the Department of Health and Human Services, and they are the best, most up-to-date advice from nutrition scientists:

1. Eat a variety of foods.
2. Maintain a healthy weight.
3. Choose a diet low in fat, saturated fat, and cholesterol.
4. Choose a diet with plenty of vegetables, fruits, and grain products.
5. Use sugars only in moderation.
6. Use salt and sodium only in moderation.
7. If you drink alcoholic beverages, do so in moderation.

Perhaps the most important—and most enjoyable—of these is "eat a variety of foods." For good health you need more than forty nutrients, and these nutrients should come from a variety of foods, not from just a few fortified foods or supplements. Choosing from the five food groups—breads and cereals; fruits; vegetables; milk; meat, poultry, and fish, and meat alternates—with moderate selections of fats and sugars, is the best way to assure variety *and* enjoy a nutritious diet as well.

▲▲

The Pyramid displays the information in the Food Guide in one symbol. And at a glance the Pyramid will help everyone to understand more about the foods they need, from which groups and in what amounts. For example, the Pyramid clearly shows that fats, oils, and sweets should be eaten sparingly—not eliminated entirely. It's an exaggeration to think that *any* food should be cut out of the diet. Some fat is essential to a healthy diet, and moderation is the message.

The three essentials of a healthy diet—proportion (or balance), moderation, and variety—are also clearly conveyed by the Pyramid. In relation to the Food Guide Pyramid, you might want to keep in mind that the USDA is quite specific about the meaning of these concepts. **Proportion** is the relative amount of food to choose from each major food group. **Moderation** is eating fats, oils, and sugars sparingly; while **variety** emphasizes the importance of eating a selection of different foods from each of the major food groups every day.

No graphic is perfect. Certainly no symbol can teach all the messages of good nutrition, and that was recognized by the USDA from the start. When it was tested, the Pyramid was found to communicate less overall misinformation than any other graphic. It was most effective in conveying those messages of proportionality, moderation, and variety.

Food guides have been around for a long time. For just over a hundred years the USDA has given Americans advice about what to eat. The USDA issued the first tables of food composition and dietary standards for the United States' population in 1894. They represented what was believed to be the average protein and calorie needs of man. Specifications were not given for vitamins and minerals, since these needs were unknown.

A few years later W. O. Atwater, a pioneer nutrition investigator with the USDA, expressed concern in a Farmer's Bulletin about obesity and the "evils of overeating." He emphasized the same themes of variety, balance, and moderation that are important to us today.

Over the years additional guides were issued as the knowledge of nutrition and of individual nutritional needs grew. Several of the guides came in response to economic constraints of the Depression and war. The first Recommended Dietary Allowances (RDAs) from the Food and Nutrition Board of the National Academy of Sciences (NAS) listed specific recommendations for calories and nine essential nutrients—protein, iron, calcium, vitamins A and D, thiamine, riboflavin, niacin, and ascorbic acid (vitamin C)—at a time when this country was at the brink of war and coping with rationing. In 1946, the USDA illustrated its food guide with a segmented circle that identified the basic seven food groups.

In the years following the war, the "Basic Seven" was revised and a new publication was issued: the *National Food Guide*. Later, in 1956, yet another new food guide, describing the "Basic Four"—was released as a booklet called *Food for Fitness—A Daily Food Guide*.

When the Senate Select Committee on Nutrition and Human Needs issued the *Dietary Goals for the United States* in 1977 a new direction was taken. This time the committee set quantitative goals for intakes of protein, carbohydrate, fat, fatty acids, cholesterol, sugars, and sodium. There were some basic disagreements, however, regarding the usual food patterns in the country. The 1977 guidelines, therefore, were not adopted by the USDA as a foundation for new food plans and food guides. In 1979, the USDA published *The Hassle-Free Guide to a Better Diet* in a colorful booklet called *Food*. The focal point of the guide was the addition of a fifth food group—fat, sugars, and alcohol—and the need to control the intake of these foods, which contribute mostly calories but few other nutrients. The guide also gave distinctive attention to calories and dietary fiber.

Though there was strong interest in health and nutrition in the late 1970s, *The Hassle-Free Guide* went unnoticed by a good many people. In 1980, the first edition of *Nutrition and Your Health: Dietary Guidelines for Americans* was issued by the USDA and the Department of Health and Human Services (DHHS). These guidelines were meant for healthy Americans, not for individuals with medical problems or who required special diets. Two revisions have been made since 1980 and the last set was issued in 1990.

In 1984, the USDA, in cooperation with the American National Red Cross, developed the "Food Wheel" as part of a consumer nutrition education course. The Food Wheel emphasized the importance of eating different amounts of food from each of the food groups. Later, in 1988, when participants in focus groups were asked to comment on the Food Wheel, they perceived it as unimaginative and old-fashioned or as providing information they already knew. Even many professionals were still under the impression that the USDA was still using the "Basic Four." Many of them didn't feel that the Food Wheel clearly addressed nutritional concerns like the intake of too much food or the connections between diet and health. A new graphic to illustrate those messages was definitely in order.

The USDA developed the Food Guide Pyramid with some explicit goals in mind. Since the Department of Agriculture spends about 60 percent of its budget on food assistance, it felt the obligation to teach proper diet and its relationship to good health to those at risk. The Dietary Guidelines were the guiding premise for the new visual. But the promotion of overall health and well-being was a prime concern. If the new guide was to be consistent with the Dietary Guidelines it would have to establish the principles of a diet for healthy Americans over two years of age that might improve and maintain overall health. The guide might also help to reduce the risk of major diet-related diseases. The graphic had to be understood by a wide range of audiences, especially children and low-income, low-literacy adults.

To be useful to consumers, foods were grouped in ways that were familiar, either from other food guides or from common knowledge. For instance, though tomatoes are technically a fruit, most people call them a vegetable; so they were kept on the vegetable list. It's worth noting that food groups in the Food Guide Pyramid were arranged with foods of similar *nutrient* content. The foods in the milk group are meant to provide calcium primarily while the foods in the meat group are primarily supplying protein. (This grouping differs from other plans, like the Diabetic Food Exchanges, where some cheeses count as a protein, or some starchy vegetables count as a bread exchange.)

One of the most notable things to me as a nutritionist is that the USDA did not want to prohibit the selection of any particular food; they wanted the guide to accommodate all types of foods. This is in line with what I've been teaching and writing about for years. It is what many dietitians espouse as the "no 'good' foods or 'bad' foods" concept. The USDA reasoned that any guide that rigidly forbids certain foods is not likely to be followed, so it's better to let consumers decide for themselves which foods they prefer as sources of fat and added sugars, instead of rigorously forbidding them. Instead of dictating that milk choices must always be nonfat, the guide would be flexible enough to show consumers how to balance a high-fat dessert, like a rich ice cream, with lower-fat selections in other food groups, so that *overall* a healthful diet was followed.

The food guide also had to account for needs that vary according to age, sex, and activity level. It was a tough challenge to create a guide that would allow varying individual nutritional needs to be met by different amounts of foods from the same groups or the same menus. That's why there are *ranges* in the number of servings from each food group. As an individual, you can determine how much of the various foods to eat based on your own age, activity level, and so forth.

Once the basic goals were established, the actual development of the new food guide began, much of it based on research that took about three years to generate and document. The Dietary Guidelines for Americans and the recommendations of several other authoritative groups were used to determine acceptable amounts of some foods, like fat and added sugars. RDAs were used to establish nutritional criteria for calories, protein, vitamins, and minerals. Previous food consumption surveys and major reports on the health and nutritional status of the population from NAS and DHHS were reviewed. Appropriate calorie ranges were set at 1,300 to 3,000 per day. Finally, it was suggested that people eat a variety of foods within the food groups to help ensure that they get enough of the nutrients for which there is no current RDA or about which little is yet known.

The biggest difference between the Food Pyramid and other food guides is the Pyramid's emphasis upon the separation of foods high in fat and added sugars but low in nutrient density. The intention was to stress the need for moderate intakes of these foods—not to eliminate them.

Then came the task of specifying *serving sizes*. Because the main message about fats, oils, and sweets is to "use sparingly," no actual serving sizes for these foods were stipulated. But the recommendation remained that only 30 percent of the calories an individual consumes should come from fat. For the other food groups a combination of factors were considered. The typical serving sizes that had been reported in the food consumption surveys were used. Serving sizes that had been listed in previous food guides were considered because people were already somewhat familiar with them. Where the two were not consistent, the traditional serving sizes that had been used in nutrition education materials (like 1 slice of bread, or ½ cup of cooked cereal) won out. The nutrient content of foods was also important. For example, foods in the milk group were looked at in terms of their calcium content; then serving sizes with approximately the equivalent amount of calcium for various foods were supplied.

When it came to the *number of servings* for each food group, specifying *ranges* for the number of servings per day was the best way to allow for calorie and nutrient needs that vary so much, depending on age, sex, activity level, and other factors. That's why six to eleven servings is the recommendation for the bread group, for instance. An active teenage boy certainly has different nutrient needs than a thirty-year-old female. The greater numbers of servings are for people with higher calorie and nutrient needs like teenage boys and very active men and women, while the lower number of servings might suit most inactive men and women and some older adults.

Companies such as Campbell's Soup, Kellogg's, and McDonald's have developed nutrition education programs, and packaging and advertising that teach and promote the philosophy of the Food Guide Pyramid. Educational packages have been and continue to be developed and distributed to USDA program directors, Cooperative Extension Service leaders, consumer and health education professionals, teachers, the media, and the food industry.

Let's move on and have a look at each of the layers of the Pyramid.

▲▲

LOOKING AT THE LAYERS

THE BREAD, CEREAL, RICE, AND PASTA GROUP

The message of the Pyramid is that eating foods from *all* of the groups, in combination with each other, is important to health. It's clear from the shape of the Pyramid that we should be getting most of our daily calories from bread, cereal, rice, and pasta. This group is also known as the Grain Group because the foods in it are made from grains.

Grains are important because they provide complex carbohydrates. Starchy foods like potatoes, pasta, rice, bread, tortillas, etc., are made up of very large, or "complex," molecules of carbohydrate. They take longer to be digested, so they provide energy for a longer, more sustained period of time than do "simple" carbohydrates. That's why complex carbohydrates are often touted for runners and other athletes who need energy and endurance. "Simple" carbohydrates like fruit or candy are digested rapidly and provide sudden, short bursts of energy. If you've ever experienced—or heard about—a "sugar rush" after eating candy or lots of high-sugar foods, it's the result of the quick breakdown of simple carbohydrates. Most complex carbohydrates are quite low in fat and also provide vitamins, minerals, and fiber. It's the fiber that makes these foods filling.

Unfortunately there is a misconception floating around that starchy foods are fattening. Nothing could be further from the truth. Starches provide only 4 calories

The Food Guide Pyramid

A Guide to Daily Food Choices

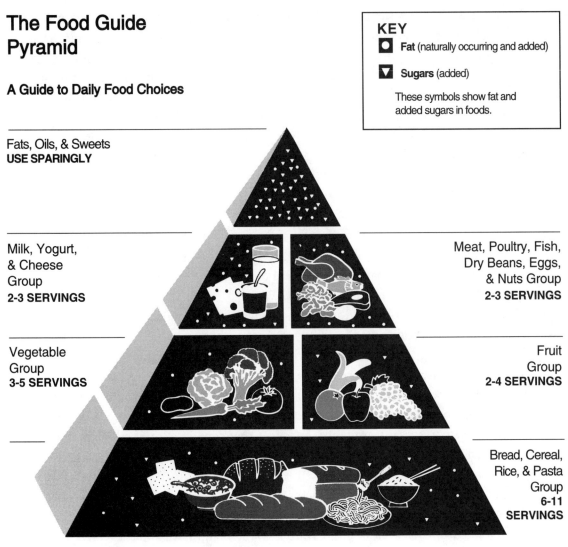

Fats, Oils, & Sweets
USE SPARINGLY

Milk, Yogurt, & Cheese Group
2-3 SERVINGS

Meat, Poultry, Fish, Dry Beans, Eggs, & Nuts Group
2-3 SERVINGS

Vegetable Group
3-5 SERVINGS

Fruit Group
2-4 SERVINGS

Bread, Cereal, Rice, & Pasta Group
6-11 SERVINGS

Source: U.S. Department of Agriculture/U.S. Department of Health and Human Services

per gram, while fats provide 9 calories per gram. It's what you, I, restaurants, food manufacturers, etc., *add* to these foods that makes them fattening. For example, potatoes are low in calories and have a fair amount of fiber. But a twice-baked potato—made with butter, cream, sour cream, and topped off with cheese—that we order in a restaurant is loaded with fat and calories. Pasta is another low-fat, high-carbohydrate choice. The sauces on pasta are often made with lots of butter, oil, and cream—that's what makes the overall dish fattening. The trick is to learn new ways to prepare low-fat sauces that are filled with flavor and equally enjoyable.

There are more nutrients in the Grain Group than most people realize. If cereals and grains are not too refined, they can be a good source of iron, zinc, vitamin B_6, thiamine, niacin, and riboflavin. Many cereals, breads, and grains are "enriched," meaning that some or all of the nutrients (vitamins and minerals) lost during processing are replaced by the manufacturer. Some of these foods are also "fortified," which means vitamins, minerals, and sometimes protein that are not in the food naturally are added. Breakfast cereals with added vitamins and minerals are an example of fortified foods.

A Word About Selection

▲ Choose several kinds of foods to get your quota from the Grain Group. Select hot or cold cereals, rice, barley, crackers, whole-grain breads, pasta, white or sweet potatoes, and vary your choices for lots of variety.

▲ Avoid coated cereals and instant hot cereals that contain a lot of sugar, and sometimes a lot of sodium.

▲ Buy whole grains and less-refined breads, cereals, and grains to get the most fiber and nutrients for your money.

▲ Select foods that are made with less fat and sugar when possible. Breadsticks, tortillas, pita bread, and popcorn are some good choices.

▲ Go easy on spreads, toppings, or sauces that contain a lot of oil or fat.

▲ Review the chapter "What's a Serving?" for more ideas on what to choose.

Freshness is also an important factor in grains, though most have a long shelf life and store well. Older grains will absorb more liquid than fresh grains, and fresh grains will cook a bit faster, require less water, and have a nuttier flavor than their elders. Quick-cooking brown rice is so much better than quick white rice. With quick-cooking barley and couscous now available, there's no reason not to try lots of different grains frequently. Even if you're an old-fashioned cook, the newly fashioned pressure cookers cook regular grain varieties faster than any other method.

Rice, pasta, potatoes, tortillas, bagels, rolls, oatmeal, couscous, hamburger buns, crackers, and pretzels are but a few of the foods from which we can choose in this layer. It forms the base of the Pyramid. Likewise these foods should form the base of daily meals and snacks.

THE FRUIT GROUP AND VEGETABLE GROUP

Fruits and vegetables appear on the next level (above Bread, Cereal, Rice, and Pasta) of the Pyramid. Though the level is divided into two sections, one for the Fruit Group and one for the Vegetable Group, we generally look at them together since they provide similar nutrients. (More information is also in the "5 a Day" chapter, page 25.)

Fruits and vegetables have lots to offer: they are high in fiber and naturally low in fat and sodium. Significant amounts of beta carotene, vitamin A, and vitamin C, along with potassium, magnesium, iron, and sometimes calcium, also come from fruits and vegetables. The Food Guide Pyramid suggests two to four servings of fruits and three to five servings of vegetables each day. Different varieties of fruits and vegetables provide different nutrients, another reason to opt for variety.

Green, leafy vegetables are good sources of beta carotene, vitamin C, calcium, and iron. Some people think that spinach and Romaine lettuce covers this category, but there's lots more to choose from in the greens family. Since they are so important, and so often overlooked, I have singled them out with some detailed information. Winter squashes are excellent sources of beta carotene, vitamin A, and fiber, but not enough people enjoy them. So I've given you some additional highlights for those as well. Many supermarket produce sections put recipe sheets and new ideas for preparation close to, or next to, vegetables. Some suppliers, like Frieda's (see page 227), even put recipe tags and decals right on the vegetable.

Remember that *variety* is always the key word. Mix-and-match your fruits as often as you can. Take a minute right now to flip over to the "5 a Day" chapter and remind yourself about all the different kinds of fruits and vegetables from which to choose. Sometimes I suggest that people eat by color: that means selecting fruits and vegetables that are yellow, green, orange, pink, and white. You'll be sure to get a wide array of nutrients that way.

Go for the Greens

Not many of us eat as much kale, collards, mustard, turnip, or beet greens as we should. If we do, it tends to be in traditional southern recipes laden with salt pork, bacon, and other fat. Instead of looking for new, lower-fat ways to prepare greens, the folks who were eating them in the first place often just abandon them altogether.

Let's take a look at greens and why we should be eating them. We'll focus on six, because they're the ones you're likely to see most often in the supermarket. They are beet greens, collards, dandelion greens, kale, mustard greens, and turnip greens. You may also find Swiss chard, sorrel, and watercress. All of them are loaded with vitamins and minerals. Beta carotene, vitamins A and C, iron, potassium, and calcium are the most notable nutrients found in greens. They are also low in calories— ranging from about 18 calories per half cup for beet greens to about 39 calories per half cup for kale—and high in fiber.

We often hear about the "cruciferous"—or cabbage—family of vegetables and how they might help prevent cancer. Some of the greens like collards and kale belong to that family, while others, like turnip greens, are simply the tops of root vegetables.

Greens have a characteristic "bite," which may range from earthy to peppery. Collards and dandelion greens, for instance, are milder when compared to turnip and mustard greens, which are quite sharp. Experiment with a few varieties to find your favorites. By all means combine several; mixing the mild and the sharp may provide just the contrast you like. Whatever you come up with, there are a few basics that are applicable to all greens.

SELECTION: Look for deep green leaves that are fresh, tender and aren't fading, yellowing, or blemished. Usually the small, young leaves are the most tender.

STORING: Lightly wrap unwashed greens in damp paper towels and put them in a plastic bag. Puncture a few holes in the bag to allow some air to flow in and refrigerate. Delicate beet greens will last for several days, while the denser ones like collards will keep for up to a week.

PREPARATION: Wash and rinse greens thoroughly. Tear out and discard tough stems or center ribs, then wash, wash, wash, using cold water and making sure to remove hidden dirt clinging to the underside of the leaves. Drain the leaves thoroughly and pat them dry. If you plan to cook them in the microwave, it is not necessary to dry them; the water that just clings to the leaves is all that's needed to cook most greens, except perhaps tougher collards, which do need a bit more water. Cut or tear the leaves into whatever size is appropriate for your recipe.

COOKING: Greens can be boiled, steamed, or microwaved. The tender ones like beet greens or young mustard greens can also be stir-fried; dandelion greens are actually best served raw. Greens can be pressure-cooked but they lose their vibrant green color, turning a drab olive green, and become bitter. Cooking time for each will vary, but all greens should be just tender to the bite. Try serving hot cooked greens with a touch of lemon juice, wine vinegar, cider vinegar, or my favorite, rice vinegar, which adds a touch of sweetness.

SEASONS: Greens are available in one form or another just about all year long. Look for collards, dandelion greens, kale, and mustard greens January through April; beet greens June through October; and turnip greens October through March.

Squash Sampler

Another category of vegetables that tends to get overlooked is the squashes. Hard-shelled squash are so outstanding that I think they deserve some special mention. They are seriously underutilized and have much to offer.

Once upon a time, hard-shelled squashes were available only in the fall and winter; we used to call them winter squash. Thanks to shrewd marketers and specialty produce companies like Frieda's (see page 227) a variety of these nutrient-filled vegetables are available just about all year round.

Hard-shelled squash—as opposed to summer squash like zucchini and yellow squash—are rich in beta carotene, high in vitamin C, and a good source of niacin, phosphorus, and potassium. They are also low in calories and sodium—a one-cup serving (cooked) has about 90 to 130 calories and less than 1 milligram of sodium—and are loaded with fiber. Best of all, this vegetable is incredibly delicious. Hard-shelled squash can be stored in a cool, dry place for months at a time.

The hard-shelled beauties come in all colors, shapes, and sizes. Their interior flesh, or pulp, also varies in color and texture. My all-time favorite squash is Kabocha, a dark green Japanese squash with a bright orange flesh that is exceptionally dense, creamy, and sweet.

If there's any shortcoming to this sublime category it is that they are definitely difficult to cut, often leaving people frustrated in their efforts to enjoy them. Read on; there's a solution to this dilemma.

A sharp vegetable knife and the microwave oven are the able assistants to make the task effortless. It was when I wrote my microwave cookbook that I became truly enamored with hard-shelled squash. When I discovered I could cook a hubbard or butternut squash in ten to twelve minutes instead of fifty to sixty minutes I was sold. It is imperative that you pierce the squash in a few places *before* you place it in the microwave so it doesn't explode. The puncture gives the steam that builds up inside the squash a place to go. And believe me, when it comes to hard-shelled squash a few pricks with a knife are a lot easier than trying to cut or slice this uncooked vegetable. Depending on what the squash is to be used for, I sometimes precook the squash just a bit in the microwave to make it easier to handle. If I want chunks for a stew, for instance, I might just heat it on HIGH for two minutes, let it stand for another minute, and then cut, slice, or dice it for the recipe. If it's for a soup, or a side-dish purée, I'll let the squash cook for ten minutes in the microwave, turning it once during cooking, then letting it stand again for one to two minutes before cutting.

Squashes vary according to the thickness of their skin and the size of the seed cavity, but generally you can figure on squash yielding the following amounts:

> 1 pound peeled, trimmed squash = about 2 cups cooked squash
> 2½ pounds whole squash = about 2 pounds cut-up
> 2 pounds untrimmed squash = about 4 servings

On a final note, don't forget about the seeds. Many squash, like pumpkin or Delicata, have edible seeds that can be rinsed and toasted either in the microwave or a conventional oven.

Here are my Top Ten Favorite Squashes for you to start sampling:

ACORN: Also known as Danish or Des Moines Table Queen, this ribbed, oval-shaped squash is generally deep green though it sometimes develops an orange color during storage. It is sweet tasting, somewhat dry, with a golden orange flesh.

AUSTRALIAN BLUE: This squatty squash has a deep bluish-green skin and a very solid exterior. It has a rich, sweet flavor and deep orange flesh.

BUTTERNUT: An elongated shape with a bulbous end and a tan color are the characteristics of this squash. It has a creamy, mildly sweet, and bright orange flesh.

CHAYOTE: This pear-shaped squash has a green or white skin that can be peeled like an apple. It is also known as a mirliton or mango squash. The mild flavor is a cross between an apple and a cucumber. It has a large, inedible seed in the center.

DELICATA: Also known as sweet potato or Bohemian squash, it has an elongated shape with longitudinal grooves. It is mildly sweet with a light texture. The green-and-tan–striped skin gives way to very tender, yellow flesh.

GOLDEN NUGGET: This small, round squash is orange-colored with ridges and resembles a tiny pumpkin. The flesh is also bright orange with a slightly sweet taste. It is a perfect single-serving squash.

KABOCHA: This Japanese variety is a round and slightly flat squash. It has a firm, deep green exterior that covers a very dense, sweet flesh that has a hearty squash flavor. It, too, has deep orange-colored pulp.

SPAGHETTI: This variety actually falls between a winter and summer squash. It has a semisoft bright yellow shell and a stringy yellow interior that separates into spaghettilike strands when cooked. The flavor is sweet and mild, with a slightly crunchy texture.

SWEET DUMPLING: A smaller version of the Delicata, it has the same round, squatty shape, and tan color with deep green streaks. It is mildly sweet with a lighter texture than some squash. The pulp is yellow-orange.

TURBAN: An intriguing vegetable that bears a striking resemblance to the headpiece of the same name, this is a somewhat flattened round squash with three top knobs. It is usually bright orange striped with cream, green, or white. The interior has a rich squash flavor and a bright orange color.

A Word About Selection

▲ Eat whole fruits as often as possible; they are excellent sources of fiber.

▲ Choose canned fruits that are packed in their own juice to avoid extra sugar.

▲ Count only 100 percent fruit juice as fruit. Beverages such as fruit "drinks," punches, cocktails, etc., contain mostly sugar and little or no fruit juice. Grape and orange sodas do not count as fruit juice.

▲ Eat dark green leafy vegetables and deep orange-colored fruits and vegetables several times a week. They are good sources of vitamins and minerals.

▲ Use low-fat salad dressings and sauces whenever possible.

There are so many fruits and vegetables to choose from that getting the recommended number of servings is hardly a chore. Salad bars in supermarkets, delicatessens, and restaurants offer a wide variety of both. Fresh fruits and vegetables have the highest nutrient values unless they have been improperly handled or have been stored too long. After three days in the supermarket and three days in your refrigerator, fresh green beans, for example, retain 41 percent *less* vitamin C than frozen green beans. Vitamin C is locked in by freezing. You should also know that frozen vegetables such as broccoli and carrots contain the same amount of vitamin A as their fresh counterparts. Use less water and reduce the cooking time for frozen vegetables so that they are tender-crisp, not soggy. When prepared this way, they are great to toss in stir-frys, soups, and sauces, and to extend pasta, rice, or meat dishes when unexpected guests arrive.

Don't overlook some of the canned varieties of fruits and vegetables either. Fruits hold up especially well in canning, and many are now packed in their own juice instead of heavy sugar syrups. Many vegetables—especially tomatoes and tomato sauces—are packed with less salt, or with "no salt added" to reduce their sodium content. Though juices have less fiber than their whole-fruit cousins they can supply the full array of nutrients available in the Fruit and Vegetable Group.

THE MILK, CHEESE, AND YOGURT GROUP

It really is true that we never outgrow our need for milk. That's because the best sources of calcium in the American diet are milk, cheese, and yogurt. More than that, the Milk—or Dairy—Group also provides protein, riboflavin, vitamins B_{12} and A, thiamine, and (when fortified) vitamin D.

The Food Guide Pyramid suggests two to three servings of milk, yogurt, and cheese per day. Two servings is suitable for most people, though women who are pregnant or breastfeeding need three servings. Teenagers and young adults—up to age twenty-four—also need three servings.

The Milk Group mainly serves to meet the nutritional need for calcium. Though people often ask me about counting some dairy foods, like cheese, as a protein equivalent I remind them that the USDA's concern is the calcium needs of the entire population. When it comes to calcium, dairy products are the primary source. It's well-known that calcium is important for building strong bones and teeth in children; it's equally important in helping to maintain the bones of adults. When bones weaken and lose their density, osteoporosis is the result.

The trick in this group is to get the nutrients, but avoid the fat (which is saturated) contained in many of the foods. Luckily, new milk, cheese, and yogurt products come in lower-fat and nonfat varieties. Some people also have trouble digesting milk—and other dairy products—but there are ways around that too. Drink or eat a small amount at a time. Buy milk to which lactase (the enzyme that

▲▲

YOGURT: MORE THAN JUST CULTURE

Yogurt deserves some special attention. You already know its place on the Pyramid. Here are some other interesting points.

- ▲ One cup (a serving) of low-fat yogurt provides adults with about 52 percent of the daily requirement for calcium; nonfat yogurt provides about 57 percent because of the added nonfat milk solids used to replace the fat.
- ▲ Yogurt also has a nice profile for vitamins B_1 and B_2 (thiamine and riboflavin), vitamin B_{12}, phosphorus, and potassium.
- ▲ Nonfat yogurt contains about 12 grams of protein per serving, and because it is an animal protein it is not only complete (lacking no amino acids) but it will also boost the value of plant proteins, which are incomplete (lacking in some amino acids), eaten during the day.
- ▲ When the yogurt is a nonfat variety that also means no cholesterol—a double bonus.
- ▲ Heat yogurt carefully when cooking it, or when adding to sauces and soups, etc. It may "break down" and curdle if it is cooked too long or at too high a temperature. If you're making a mustard sauce, for instance, remove the pan from the heat before whisking in the yogurt.
- ▲ Use yogurt as a substitute for mayonnaise or sour cream in salad dressings, soups, sauces, desserts, muffins, or cheese (see page 65). But do it judiciously, especially in the beginning. Yogurt does have its own distinctive tang that, for some people, takes some getting accustomed to. Start out with a half-and-half replacement in the beginning and move along from there.

▲▲

breaks down milk sugar—lactose) has been added. You can also buy LactAid in drug or health food stores, in liquid, powder, or tablet form, which you can add to foods on your own.

While we're on the subject of dairy foods, yogurt deserves some special mention. Though yogurt has grown immensely in popularity in this country, many people still don't realize just how versatile it can be. Yogurt is a readily portable form of milk. It's a food that can be eaten right out of the carton as a snack, or as part of a quick meal on the run. What's even better is that yogurt is, almost always, a dairy product that many people who cannot otherwise tolerate milk products can easily digest.

Live active cultures, or "friendly" bacteria, give yogurt its special taste and custardy texture, and also enhance its digestibility. That is why people who are lactose intolerant—or who have difficulty digesting milk and other dairy products—often are able to eat yogurt. Yogurt also eases the digestion of casein, an important protein in milk.

Recent studies indicate that yogurt may offer more than just nutritive value. Yogurt, it seems, helps to prevent and combat digestive tract infections. Live active cultures have the ability to flourish in the digestive tract, where they can have a natural antibiotic effect. The cultures secrete lactic acid and other substances that may help

▲▲

SEE FOR YOURSELF: HOW YOGURT STACKS UP

(PER ONE-CUP SERVING)

	CALORIES	CALCIUM (MG)	FAT (G)	CHOLESTEROL (MG)
Nonfat plain yogurt	110	452	.5	5
Low-fat plain yogurt	140	415	4	15
Whole-milk plain yogurt	140	274	7	29
Sour cream	415	225	40	80
Light sour cream	290	—	20	60
Mayonnaise	1,585	30	176	130
Cottage cheese (2%)	203	154	4	18
Heavy cream	830	160	90	335

▲▲

combat harmful gastrointestinal organisms that can cause such conditions as diarrhea and food poisoning. It takes decades of carefully designed and repeated studies to confirm results, but preliminary studies indicate that yogurt can help to boost the immune system and that yogurt may be useful in lowering serum (blood) cholesterol.

To be sure you get the most benefits from yogurt, check that the label says: "live and active yogurt cultures," "living yogurt cultures," or "contains active cultures."

A Word About Selection

▲ Choose skim milk and nonfat yogurt as often as possible; they are the lowest in fat. It may take a little time to get used to the taste and texture of skim milk. Try mixing it with some regular milk and gradually increase the portion of skim milk.

▲ Remember that cottage cheese is lower in calcium than most cheeses. One cup of cottage cheese counts as a half serving of milk. There is a wide assortment of low sodium, low-fat and nonfat, fruit, and vegetable cottage cheeses from which to choose. Cottage cheese also makes a nice ingredient for casseroles, lasagnas, and baked goods.

▲ Some of the hard cheeses like cheddar and Swiss are usually very high in saturated fats and sodium. There are some low-fat and low-sodium ones available, and some definitely taste better than others. You may need to taste a few to find one you like (see "Supermarkets Get Savvy," page 191).

▲ Ice milk and frozen yogurt can be counted as a serving. They often contain a lot of added sugar, so choose them in moderation.

It's important to stress that people who do not drink milk or eat dairy products should check with a registered dietitian or physician to get help planning ways to get enough calcium. This is especially important for children, teens, women who are pregnant or breastfeeding, and anyone at risk for osteoporosis.

Some other foods provide calcium. Dark green leafy vegetables like broccoli, spinach, collards, and kale are sources of calcium. Canned fish, like sardines and salmon, have soft, edible bones that are rich in calcium. Tortillas made with cornmeal fortified with calcium can help fill your quota too. The Dairy Group, however, is the most important and the best source of dietary calcium. You don't want to skimp on it.

▲▲

WORK IN SOME CALCIUM

Creative boosters can help folks of all ages get the calcium they need. Try these, which don't require much effort.

- ▲ Add powdered nonfat dry milk to muffins, breads, and casseroles.
- ▲ Crumble tofu, a soy product that is sometimes made with calcium sulfate (check the label) on top of salads, chilis, and stews; purée it for salad dressings, and add it crumbled or cubed to stir-frys.
- ▲ Use skim or low-fat milk to make soups, casseroles, puddings, pancake batters, and milkshakes.
- ▲ Make salad dressings, sauces, and dips with nonfat yogurt.

▲▲

THE MEAT, POULTRY, FISH, DRY BEANS, EGGS, AND NUTS GROUP

Protein is the main nutrient that this segment of the Pyramid is meant to deliver. Iron, zinc, and the B vitamins—especially B_{12}—are also supplied from the animal products: beef, pork, lamb, poultry, game, and seafood. Other foods in this group—dry beans, peas, and nuts—are similar to meat in terms of the protein they provide. They also add a significant amount of fiber, but they lack vitamin B_{12}.

Iron is an important nutrient found in many foods, but its best sources are meat, poultry, and fish. Dried beans and peas (whole-grain cereals and dark green leafy vegetables too) are also significant sources of iron. The iron in these plant foods, however, is in a form that is not as well absorbed by the body as the iron in meat, poultry, and fish. Eating a vitamin C–rich food along with them in a meal or a snack is a good way to increase the amount of iron the body absorbs. You can also combine a small amount of meat, poultry, or fish to enhance the iron absorption from plant foods.

From this group, a total of 5 to 7 ounces, or two to three servings a day, is recommended for adults. Count 2 to 3 ounces of cooked lean meat, poultry, or fish as a serving. For those who are vegetarians, or want an occasional meatless meal, substitute the following for 1 ounce of meat: one-half cup of cooked beans; 2 tablespoons of peanut butter; 4 ounces of tofu; one-quarter cup of seeds; or one-third cup of nuts. Whatever you choose, it's a good idea to make selections that are lean and low in fat to stay within the recommendation of deriving only 30 percent of daily calories from fat. Peanut butter, nuts, and seeds are high in fat, so use them in moderation. Dried beans, peas, and lentils make a better trade-off because they are high in fiber and virtually fat-free.

The fat and cholesterol content of meats varies widely. Generally there tends to be less of both in game, poultry, and fish. But that is changing: farmers are now raising livestock to be leaner, and leaner choices at the meat counter are available on a regular basis. Veal is higher in cholesterol than other beef products, but lower in *total* fat content because these younger animals have not yet developed as much fat tissue. Even if you are watching cholesterol, there's no reason not to have veal occasionally. Overall, selecting lower-fat cuts of meat and avoiding rich, high-fat sauces and gravies is the best way to keep your fat and cholesterol under control.

Though other meal plans may exchange some cheese for protein servings, the Food Guide Pyramid does not. Remember the framework here is the provision of protein, B vitamins, and zinc—cheeses don't meet this requirement. Save them for your calcium quotas.

A Word About Selection

▲ Choose lean cuts of meats that include round, loin, sirloin, and chuck arm beef; all cuts of veal except ground; leg, loin, and fore shanks of lamb; light and dark meat of turkey and chicken (eaten without the skin); and fish and shellfish that are low in fat (most are, but avoid fatty ones like bluefish, for instance, or fish canned in oil).

▲ Prepare meats and fish in trim and tasty ways: broil, roast, stir-fry, steam, and poach instead of frying. Use a microwave oven, pressure cooker, or slow cooker (Crock-Pot) to reduce the fat and retain the flavor.

▲ Processed meats such as hot dogs, bacon, salami, and bologna are high in fats and sodium. Limit them to an occasional selection.

▲ Use eggs and egg yolks moderately. That does *not* mean you must eliminate eggs from your diet. The American Heart Association says that most people may safely eat about three eggs per week. You may want to substitute two whites for one whole egg when baking recipes call for several eggs.

▲ Include nuts and seeds only occasionally. They do have lots of fiber but are high in fat.

▲ Try more game meats like rabbit and venison, which are lower in fat than most meats.

▲ Include more dry beans and peas in recipes; and look for dishes that include them when ordering in a restaurant.

FATS, OILS, AND SWEETS

The small tip of the Pyramid may actually represent the majority of calories for many Americans. The goal of the Food Guide Pyramid is to change that. Foods such as salad dressings and oils, cream, butter, margarine, sugars, soft drinks, candies, and sweet desserts provide calories but offer little else from a nutritional point of view. You don't need to eliminate any of them from your meals and snacks, but some moderation is certainly in order.

This is the time to mention, by the way, that alcoholic beverages fall in this segment of the Pyramid because calories are just about all they provide. Because the Food Pyramid is fashioned after the U.S. Dietary Guidelines, the same "If you drink, do so in moderation" concept holds true.

Keeping total fat to 30 percent of the daily calories is the message of the Pyramid. Most of the time you can easily do this by merely making lower-fat choices in the foods you are currently eating, and avoiding "extras" like sauces, toppings, and gravies. In general, foods that come from animals (milk and meat products) are higher in fat than foods that come from plants. But with all the low-fat meat and low- and nonfat dairy choices available, no favorite foods need to be given up altogether.

Fat has more than twice the calories per gram than either carbohydrate or protein. Fat has 9 calories per gram, while carbohydrate and protein contain only 4 per gram. That means when you start to lower your fat intake—and reduce fat calories—it is only reasonable to replace them with other foods to maintain energy levels. This is another reason that the six to eleven servings of cereals and grains or five servings of fruits and vegetables is not extraordinary. Fats give a feeling of "satiety," or fullness, so adding fruits, vegetables, and grain products, which are naturally low in fat and high in fiber, will keep you full even though you're eating less fat.

We often talk about cholesterol and fat as if they are the same thing, but they're not. Dietary cholesterol is a fatlike substance present in all animal foods: meat, poultry, fish, milk and milk products, and egg yolks. Plant foods do not contain cholesterol. Dietary cholesterol and saturated fat (also found in animal foods) raise blood cholesterol levels in many people. That can increase their risk for heart disease. The Food Guide Pyramid agrees with many health authorities that cholesterol should be limited to an average of 300 milligrams or less per day.

A Final Note on Salt and Sodium

No, you don't have to give up salt, even though most people probably consume much more than they really need. Health authorities say that sodium intake should not be higher than 2,400 to 3,000 milligrams per day. That is the combination of salt added to foods at the table and salt and sodium that has already been added to food in processing. One teaspoon of salt, by the way, contains 2,000 milligrams of sodium.

Do try to go easy on foods that are high in sodium, like soy sauce, luncheon meats, and many cheeses. Information on food labels can help you know how much you're getting and how to make better food choices.

A Word About Fats, Oils, and Sugars

▲ Choose liquid oils instead of solid fats whenever possible.

▲ Watch out for "hidden" sugar in soft drinks, cereals, and desserts; as well as added sugars from food like chocolate milk, sorbet, gelatin desserts, and fruit canned in heavy syrup.

▲ Use low- or nonfat salad dressings whenever possible.

▲ Try to limit added sugars to around 6 teaspoons per day, if you're eating 1,600 calories; 12 teaspoons at 2,200 calories; or 18 teaspoons at 2,800 calories. Remember, added sugars include candies, soft drinks, and jams, as well as sugar added to your coffee or cereal. Please see the chart on page 24, "Where Is the Hidden Sugar?"

▲ Look for lower-salt and no-salt-added versions of food items in supermarkets.

▲ *Sugars* include all forms of caloric sweeteners including honey, molasses, white and brown sugar, and corn syrup.

▲▲▲

WHERE IS THE HIDDEN SUGAR?

There can be lots of sugar in foods and beverages other than what we add at the table. Here are some common items and the approximate amount of sugar they contain:

Fruit pie with crust (1 slice)	6 teaspoons
Fruit canned in heavy syrup (½ cup)	4 teaspoons
Low-fat fruit yogurt (8 ounces)	7 teaspoons
Chocolate milk 2% (1 cup)	3 teaspoons
Ice cream, ice milk, or frozen yogurt (½ cup)	3 teaspoons
Cereal, sugar-coated (1 cup)	5 teaspoons*
Syrup or honey (1 tablespoon)	3 teaspoons
Jam (1 tablespoon)	3 teaspoons
Soda (1 12-ounce can)	9 teaspoons
Fruit drink or ade (12 ounces)	12 teaspoons

* Check product label; some may vary. (Note: 4 grams of sugar = 1 teaspoon.)

▲▲▲

▲▲

5 A DAY

Eat more fruits and vegetables. We've all heard these words for about as long as we can remember.

The 1988 "U.S. Surgeon General's Report on Nutrition and Health" urged Americans to eat more fruits and vegetables. In March 1989, the National Academy of Sciences urged Americans to eat at least five servings each day and suggested that at least one of those servings be one that is rich in vitamin C, and one be high in vitamin A. The report also spelled out emphatically that for the two out of three adults who do not drink excessively or smoke, the single most important personal choice influencing long-term health is what they eat!

Just after that report was issued more and more research and information came out documenting that fruits and vegetables may lower the risk of several diseases. In fact, according to the National Cancer Institute, 35 percent of all cancer deaths may be related to what we eat. Diets that are high in fat and low in fiber seem to place people at greater risk not only for certain types of cancer, but also for diabetes, coronary heart disease, stroke, and atherosclerosis. Nutrition experts and major health organizations agree that the American diet contains too much fat and not enough fruits, vegetables, and whole grains.

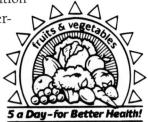

Fruits and vegetables without added fats have lots of benefits. On their own, they're low in calories, fat, and sodium. Many are good sources of nutrients like calcium,

25

iron, potassium, and folic acid. Because they're high in fiber, fruits and vegetables promote a healthy digestive tract—which means they reduce constipation.

It only took a few years after the Surgeon General's Report for the National Cancer Institute to stand behind the results of the studies that indicated the positive role of fruits and vegetables for reducing certain types of cancer. In 1991 they teamed up with the Produce for Better Health Foundation and created the 5 a Day for Better Health campaign. Their prime objective was to advance a national health objective that would increase the intake of vegetables and fruits from two and a half daily servings to five servings by the year 2000.

Initially the program started at the retail level. Grocery stores and supermarket chains were eligible to participate if they displayed the 5 a Day logo in the stores, did some advertising, and also offered brochures, food demonstrations, recipes, and other information about the storage and handling of fruits and vegetables. Eventually the program was picked up by restaurants and food companies, and incorporated into education programs used in schools.

Just as 5 a Day was getting started, a baseline survey was conducted to get an accurate picture of what people already knew about fruits and vegetables. Despite the fact that the Department of Health and Human Services, the U.S. Department of Agriculture, the National Cancer Institute, and the National Academy of Sciences have all been urging Americans to eat five servings a day or more of fruits and vegetables, only 8 percent of those surveyed knew that five or more servings are needed for good health. A full 34 percent felt that one serving or less of fruits and vegetables were what you should eat for good health, and 32 percent thought two servings a day were enough.

Older Americans were especially prone to underestimate the number of fruits and vegetables needed. Although their consumption was the highest of any group, at four servings a day, almost half (44 percent) of those age sixty-five and over thought they needed one or fewer servings per day, and three out of four thought they needed two or fewer. The lowest numbers of servings per week were among eighteen- to thirty-four-year-olds, while the highest were for those age sixty-five and over.

Women tend to eat five more servings of fruits and vegetables per week than men. Women are also more likely than men to think that a person needs a larger number of servings for good health. Almost half (45 percent) of the men said that one or fewer servings is sufficient, compared to 25 percent of women. Surprisingly, men eat less whole fruit than women.

There were some ethnic differences in the survey too. Black Americans tend to eat more fruit and juice, with an average of about four more servings a week than whites or Hispanics. Whites, however, lead in vegetable consumption, eating three more servings than blacks in an average week, and about four more than Hispanics. Fortunately 71 percent of the people who reported that they eat the least produce say they like the taste of fruits a lot, and 56 percent said they like the taste of vegetables.

The message of 5 a Day is simple: "Eat five a day for better health." Remember that within those five servings it's a good idea to target the choices so they include vitamin A, vitamin C, vegetables from the cabbage (cruciferous) family, and at least one high-fiber selection each day. You'll want to keep in mind the main sources for each:

VITAMIN A: Apricots, cantaloupe, mango, and papaya; broccoli, bok choy, carrots, kale, turnip greens, Swiss chard, beet and mustard greens, spinach, Romaine lettuce, winter squash, sweet potatoes, and tomatoes.

VITAMIN C: Oranges, grapefruit, kiwi, cantaloupe, honeydew, papaya, mango, raspberries, strawberries, and watermelon; asparagus, bok choy, broccoli, Brussels sprouts, cabbage, cauliflower, green and red bell pepper, and tomatoes.

▲▲

FIVE POINTS TO REMEMBER

The 5 a Day Program is easy to follow. Just keep in mind these five quick suggestions:

1. Eat five servings of fruits and vegetables a day.
2. Eat at least one vitamin A–rich selection every day.
3. Eat at least one vitamin C–rich selection every day.
4. Eat at least one high-fiber selection every day.
5. Eat cabbage-family (cruciferous) vegetables several times each week.

Five servings may sound like a lot to most people, but it's really not. You'll be astonished to see how little it comes out to be and how easily "servings" add up. See "One Serving Equals," page 28.

▲▲

HIGH-FIBER: Cooked dried beans and lentils are about the best, and they include black, garbanzo (chick-peas), cannellini, kidney, navy, and pinto beans. There is a multitude of "boutique" dried beans now available in gourmet stores. They come in a wide array of colors and shapes. Some of the more unusual are scarlet runners, calypso, yellow eye, black soybeans. Serving these may encourage finicky eaters to eat more legumes. Whole and split green or yellow dried peas are also high-fiber choices.

CRUCIFEROUS OR CABBAGE FAMILY: Mustard, turnip, and beet greens, kale, Swiss chard, broccoli, Brussels sprouts, bok choy, cabbage, and cauliflower are the leaders here.

▲▲

ONE SERVING EQUALS

If you think that five servings of fruits and vegetables is a lot, take a look at what counts as a serving. Chances are that your ordinary portions are equal to two or three servings. So you've got a head start already. According to the Pyramid, one serving equals:

- ▲ ½ cup fruit—cut-up frozen, fresh, and canned fruits
- ▲ ½ grapefruit
- ▲ 1 medium piece of fresh fruit such as banana, orange, or apple
- ▲ ¾ cup (or 6 ounces) of 100 percent fruit or vegetable juice
- ▲ ½ cup cooked vegetables or legumes (dried peas or beans)
- ▲ 1 medium-size raw vegetable such as a carrot or rib of celery
- ▲ 6 to 8 carrot sticks (3 inches long)
- ▲ 1 medium potato
- ▲ 1 cup raw leafy greens such as bok choy, lettuce, escarole, kale, Swiss chard, or spinach
- ▲ ¼ cup dried fruit such as prunes, raisins, apricots, dates, or figs

Note: The serving sizes for children will vary. It's best to discuss feeding them with a pediatrician or a registered dietitian. Because many children don't eat much all at once, it's a good idea to serve them smaller portions more frequently.

▲▲

Time is a pretty precious commodity to most of us these days. I often hear people complain that they only have time to shop for groceries once a week, or that they don't have a refrigerator to hold a lot, or that they often skip meals or eat on the run. These are all valid considerations in careful diet planning, though they shouldn't stop you from heeding a few pointers to solve the dilemma.

For instance if you shop once a week, or if your refrigerator is small, consider frozen or canned fruits and vegetables as a supplement to the fresh ones. Frozen items have really come a long way from some of those with which we grew up. I was quite amazed when I did a project that required using frozen vegetables. I hadn't been near the freezer case in years and I was forced to develop some recipes that used a wide variety of frozen foods. Not only was the quality and taste better than I remembered, but my guests truly raved about the dishes I served. Even items like kale, collards, yams, and small whole onions are available. Both frozen and canned vegetables are good for adding to soups, stews, and casseroles. Canned or frozen fruits are especially useful in muffins and pancakes, or puréed as a sauce. Look for vegetables that are low-sodium and fruits that are canned in their own juice.

There's no question that fresh produce in season is a good buy and a boost to good health. Fresh peaches, watermelon, carrots, and potatoes can be some of the best bargains in the supermarket, but frozen and canned fruits and vegetables can also be very economical.

If things are especially hectic, plan ahead and work in a few of your servings as snacks or quick meals. Keep dried fruits in your desk or briefcase, or tuck in some fresh fruit for eating on the train. Whirl a ripe pear, banana, or berries in a blender with some nonfat yogurt for a quick breakfast before you dash out in the morning. Even vending machines are now stocking 8-ounce containers of plain yogurt. With a piece of fruit, one of these containers makes a nutritious and easy lunch if you're traveling or eating at your desk. Consider getting an office refrigerator too. Stock it with juices; carrot, celery, cucumber, or zucchini sticks; cherry tomatoes; or any easy-to-eat finger food. Add lettuce and tomato to your sandwich or burger, have pizza with vegetables, drink pure fruit juice, and substitute a small salad with low-fat dressing for french fries. Do beware of salad bars, where often the items are premade with dressing and have been sitting in the pan and absorbing extra oil. Low-fat dressings may not always be available. Ask for a wedge of lemon when they're not, and look around for a cruet of vinegar or hot sauce that can be used instead to add flavor. Most salad bar ladles, by the way, hold up to 4 tablespoons of dressing. At 70 calories a tablespoon for regular dressings, that may be 280 calories you're dumping on your so-called "diet" lunch.

My Kids Eat Vegetables . . .

Getting kids to eat vegetables (and sometimes fruits) is the bane of almost every parent's existence. There are a few exceptions out there, but for most it's a struggle. It's not impossible though. Cooked vegetables have a much stronger flavor to children than they do to adults, so the first trick may be to offer them raw vegetables that they can eat plain or with a dip. Pepper strips—red, yellow, orange, green—are especially appealing. Carrot sticks and yellow and green (zucchini) squash sliced or cut into strips are also popular, and even though most kids refuse cooked spinach, a spinach salad can be inviting. Variety may be even more important to kids than it is to adults, and many of the same vitamins and minerals found in vegetables are also found in fruits. So if they accept fruits more readily, go for it. That means, however, melons, grapes, berries, nectarines, peaches, plums, and oranges—not just apples and bananas.

Summing It All Up

Study after study confirms that eating more fruits and vegetables plays a role in preventing many types of cancer. Two scientists at the University of Minnesota (Drs. Kristi Steinmetz and John Potter) actually reviewed 137 such studies and concluded that consuming more fruits and vegetables was consistently associated with a reduced risk of cancer. Dr. Gladys Block of the University of California at Berkeley, another noted scientist, reviewed a large number of studies comparing the intake of fruits and vegetables and the incidence of cancer. She and her colleagues noted that for most cancers, people who ate fewer fruits and vegetables were at twice the risk compared with those who consumed more of these foods.

It's important to note here that although a lot of what we see and hear relates to a single nutrient like beta carotene or vitamin C, there is, in the words of one researcher at the National Cancer Institute, "no magic bullet." In other words, it's pretty certain that nutrients in food work together and all of them are important.

▲▲

TEN WAYS TO GET 5 A DAY:

1. Sip some juice.
2. Have your low-fat frozen yogurt with berries on top.
3. Blend fresh fruit with skim milk or nonfat yogurt for a fast breakfast start.
4. Keep dried fruit like apricots, raisins, dates, and pineapple at your desk for nibbling.
5. Say yes to tomato and lettuce for your burger or sandwich.
6. Top pancakes with fruit purées, bananas, or berries.
7. Order a side vegetable as an appetizer.
8. Purée berries, mangoes, bananas, or papayas for a tasty, fat-free dessert sauce.
9. Add more fruits to savory dishes. Mandarin orange slices, kiwi, cranberries, and grapes make a nice addition to pork, fish, and poultry.
10. Freeze grapes to have on hand as a refreshing snack.

▲▲

▲▲

WHAT'S A SERVING?

It always fascinates me to watch the response of people in my weight management groups or health education workshops when I tell them the number of servings from each of the food groups in the Pyramid. Many of them just about go berserk when they hear that six to eleven servings is suggested from the Grain Group.

At first I was surprised by their reaction, and then it became clear to me that the *real* problem was that they didn't understand what a "serving" is. Once I make it clear, the commotion quiets down, and they are able to appreciate that this number of servings isn't so absurd after all.

I hope that I can clarify this point once and for all. In most cases, a serving is NOT a helping, nor is it what you are served in a restaurant, nor is it what you select from the salad bar, nor is it what comes out of a can or a single frozen dinner entrée, nor is it what Mom places in front of you at the breakfast table. A serving is a unit that has been designated by food and health professionals to represent an amount of food within a group or category, like the Meat Group or Fruit Group.

The most widely known and used serving sizes (by professionals) are probably those used in former food guides like the Basic Four. Serving sizes developed for the Pyramid consider typical serving sizes that have been reported in food consumption surveys, serving units that people can easily multiply or divide to exemplify what they have eaten, amounts with similar nutrient content within the same food group, and finally, traditional amounts that have been generally designated as a serving in past food guides. Serving sizes are meant to be guides in helping us to assess our portions and the corresponding amount of nutrients we consume.

There are many tables and references for servings in cookbooks—especially those that are geared to weight loss—and in magazine and newspaper articles. But there's more to becoming familiar with servings than just reading about them, and I find the show-and-tell method the most effective in helping people understand what a serving really is.

I often bring a set of measuring spoons, measuring cups, a food scale, and a couple of wineglasses to my nutrition classes. Then I pour and weigh a few well-known foods and beverages, and the fun begins. That large New York–style bagel you had for breakfast weighs 4 ounces, which means you've had almost four bread servings before leaving the house in the morning! One serving of rice is a half cup. When I measure that out and put it on a plate, there is no one in the group who would say they eat that small amount of rice for dinner. One cup looks more like it: that's two servings. It's pretty much the same with liquids. Few people drink less than 6 fluid ounces of wine, though the "standard drink" serving (in the Dietary Guidelines) is 5 fluid ounces, and most people drink about 6 fluid ounces of juice. That is what's called a serving.

Once this observation hits home, the impression that six to eleven servings from the Bread Group is more than they could eat in a day is overturned. Weighing and measuring, or show-and-tell, is the best way to get a handle on what a serving looks like. This lesson is worth a thousand words and lasts a lifetime. It is also enormously helpful in gauging what we're actually eating when we're in a restaurant or a friend's home.

I hope you'll try this exercise using some of your favorite foods. You may find

▲▲

WHAT A SERVING LOOKS LIKE

If weighing and measuring is not for you, there are a few visual cues you can use to estimate an approximate serving size.

- ▲ ½ cup is the size of . . . a small fist
- ▲ 1 cup is the size of . . . a small hand holding a tennis ball
- ▲ 3 ounces of meat, fish, or poultry is about the size of . . . a deck of cards

▲▲

that recommendations such as those given for the Food Pyramid, or in the 5 a Day program, turn out to be pretty easy to follow.

Here is a list of some of the common foods in each group and what counts as a serving.

GRAINS, CEREALS, BREADS, PASTA, ETC. (6–11 SERVINGS)

1 slice white, whole-wheat, unfrosted raisin, French, or Italian bread (1 ounce is a serving)

½ English muffin
½ hamburger bun
1 6-in. flour tortilla
2 breadsticks (4 in. × ½ in.)
4 rye crisps
4 saltines
½ cup cooked pasta

½ cup cooked barley
½ cup cooked whole grains
   (quinoa, bulgur, or millet)
1 ounce ready-to-eat breakfast cereal
½ cup cooked cereal
½ cup cooked rice
3 tablespoons wheat germ

FRUITS (2–4 SERVINGS)

¾ cup juice
1 medium apple, orange, or banana
½ cup mandarin oranges
2 plums
3 apricots
12 large cherries
15 grapes
½ cup sliced strawberries
½ cup blueberries
1 large kiwi
½ large or 1 small pear

½ grapefruit
½ mango or papaya
2 raw figs, 2 in. across
½ cup cooked or canned fruit
½ cup melon cubes
½ cup raspberries
½ cup blackberries
¼ cup dried fruit
½ cup fresh pineapple cubes
1 peach (2¾ in. across)

VEGETABLES (3–5 SERVINGS)

1 cup raw leafy vegetables (spinach, kale, beet greens, etc.)

½ cup nonleafy, raw, chopped vegetables

¾ cup vegetable juice

½ cup cooked beans and peas (kidney, split, blackeye)

1 ear of corn on the cob (6 in. long)

1 small baked potato (3 oz.)

½ cup cooked vegetables

½ cup cooked lentils

½ cup winter squash

½ cup green peas

½ cup corn

½ cup lima beans

½ cup sweet potato

Vary your vegetable choices to include:

Asparagus, beets, broccoli, Brussels sprouts, cabbage, carrots, cauliflower, eggplant, green beans, greens (collard, mustard, turnip), kohlrabi, leeks, mushrooms, okra, pea pods, peppers, rutabaga, spinach, summer squash, tomatoes, turnips, water chestnuts, zucchini.

MILK, YOGURT, AND CHEESE (2–3 SERVINGS)*

Teenagers, women who are pregnant or breastfeeding, and young adults to age twenty-four need three servings a day.

1 CUP:

skim milk

low-fat (1% or 2%) milk

whole milk

chocolate milk (2%)

yogurt, low-fat, plain

yogurt, nonfat, plain

yogurt, low-fat, fruit

yogurt, low-fat, flavored (lemon, vanilla, etc.)

yogurt, nonfat, flavored (lemon, vanilla, etc.)

buttermilk, low-fat

* Select low- and nonfat items whenever possible.

½ cup evaporated skimmed milk
½ cup evaporated whole milk
⅓ cup dry nonfat milk
½ cup ricotta cheese, part-skim
½ cup ricotta cheese, nonfat
2 cups cottage cheese

1½ cups ice milk
1 cup frozen yogurt
2 ounces process cheese
1½ ounces natural cheese (Cheddar, mozzarella, etc.)

MEAT, POULTRY, FISH, AND PROTEIN ALTERNATIVES (2–3 SERVINGS FOR A TOTAL OF 5–7 OUNCES)*

3 ounces lean meat, poultry, fish, cooked
(Note: a medium baked chicken breast half [flesh only] = 3 ounces cooked meat; and a drumstick [flesh only] = 1½ ounces cooked meat)
3 ounces lean ground meat, cooked
3 ounces lean game (rabbit, venison, buffalo, etc.), cooked
3 ounces fish or shellfish = 15 medium shrimp, 6 sea scallops, 6 clams, 15 small sardines
3 ounces lean sliced meat (ham, turkey, roast beef, roast lamb, etc.)
3 ounces flaked tuna

* Select low-fat items whenever possible.

PROTEIN ALTERNATIVES FOR ONE OUNCE OF MEAT:

1 egg
¼ cup egg substitute
2 tablespoons peanut butter
⅓ cup nuts

½ cup dry beans, peas, lentils, cooked
4 ounces tofu

FATS, OILS, AND SWEETS—USE SPARINGLY

Butter, margarine, mayonnaise, salad dressing, cream cheese, sour cream, whipped cream, sugar, honey, syrups, jam, cola and other soft drinks, fruit drinks like cocktails and ades, chocolate, sherbet, sorbet, and gelatin desserts are some of the higher-fat and/or sugar-laden foods we consume.

Most people say that it's easier for them to count *grams* of fat rather than fat calories. That's great because the Pyramid recommendations of limiting fat to 30 percent of daily calories can easily be translated into grams.

Use this ready-reference chart to track your fat intake.

DAILY CALORIE LEVEL	TOTAL GRAMS OF FAT	TOTAL CALORIES FROM FAT
1,000*	33	300
1,200	40	360
1,500	50	450
1,800	60	540
2,000	66	600
2,200	73	660
2,800	93	840

* This is a limited number of calories that should not be maintained for any length of time or without medical supervision.

I hope you're able to recognize that all your favorite foods can be part of a Pyramid eating plan. Cakes and cookies count in the Bread Group; a cheeseburger is a meat option plus dairy and bread; ice cream fits in with milk, yogurt, and cheese. Whenever you are eating these foods just remember to counterbalance them with lower-fat choices.

A FINAL NOTE ON THE NUMBERS

Do remember that the *range* of servings given in the Pyramid is trying to cover just about everybody. The amount of food you need depends on your age, sex, physical condition, and how active you are. Just about everybody should have *at least* the minimum number of servings from each of the food groups on a daily basis. Most men and teenagers and many women and older children need more than that. The top of the range is meant for active men, teenage boys, and athletes.

Obviously young children have smaller needs. They can have smaller servings from all the groups, except milk, which should total two servings per day. For kids ages two to four a serving can be about one-third smaller than those listed above *except* for milk. Those servings may also be spaced throughout the day, and given as snacks, rather than expecting the child to eat them all at a particular meal. Unless your child is very active, he or she probably won't want to eat too much at one time. A few tablespoons of applesauce or mashed potato may be just about right. After age six your child may be able to eat the lower numbers of full-size servings on the Pyramid. On the other hand, if the child is very active, extra servings are appropriate. Be sensitive to his or her individual needs. Even kids in the same family may have very different eating styles and requirements.

It is always wise to consult a registered dietitian if you are a vegetarian or if you have food allergies or other clinical considerations like ulcers or diabetes. Individuals who do not consume dairy products will also need special guidance on meeting their calcium needs. (Yogurt is often helpful for these people; pages 17–18 have more details.) Parents of infants and toddlers (under age two) should speak to an R.D. or the child's pediatrician for advice on feeding at this stage.

▲▲

ABOUT THE RECIPES
AND PYRAMID EQUIVALENTS

The recipes in this book were carefully developed to conform with the Pyramid and the Dietary Guidelines. My main goal was to be sure the finished recipes were delicious and flavorful—as you can tell from the subtitle of the book. It was also important that they be easy. I want people to *cook* these recipes, not to be overwhelmed or intimidated by them. So in most cases, I limited the number of ingredients. The recipes are low in fat and cholesterol and the use of salt is kept to a minimum.

Nowadays most people don't seem to have the time (or the inclination) to cook elaborate meals during the week. There are lots of "weekend chefs" who love to dabble in the kitchen for hours on Saturday and Sunday, but this book is aimed at the Monday to Friday folks. I hope you'll make the Food Pyramid part of your lives. Having recipes that are quick and practical is a good way to get started.

There's a wide variety of recipes from which to choose that should fit just about any taste or preference. Some of them are old favorites like Creamy Mashed Potatoes or Roast Chicken, while others like Greek Rabbit Stew or Venison and Red Bean Chili may be new. Everyone will enjoy the meatless main dishes here, whether or not they are vegetarians. Penne with Greens and Beans, Lasagna with Spinach and Lentils, or Black Bean Chili with Red Peppers and Corn can be served to meat eaters without the slightest hesitation.

The microwave recipes were tested in a 650-watt microwave oven with the following power settings. You may want to alter the timing on those recipes depending on the wattage of your microwave.

HIGH	100% power
MEDIUM-HIGH	70% power
MEDIUM	50% power
MEDIUM-LOW	30% power
LOW (Defrost)	10% power

A 6-quart Magafesa pressure cooker was the type I used for recipe testing. It is the latest—and perhaps quickest—cooker on the market because the seal is very tight and the pressure settings accurate. If you have an older, jiggle-top cooker you might do well to add a few minutes to the timings I suggested. In any event, don't fill your cooker more than two-thirds full for best results. (See Resources, page 225, for mail-order information.)

A Word About the Ingredients

All of the recipes were developed using ingredients that are readily available throughout the United States. Where an item is more easily found somewhere other than in the supermarket, I have added a note.

Chicken and vegetable broths are always the low-sodium variety. I strongly recommend that you make them from scratch. Not only is the flavor far superior to any that you will purchase, you are also able to control the amount of added salt (if any). I have given you salt-free recipes for both broths (pages 131 and 133). To defat stock, chill it overnight; any remaining fat will rise to the top and solidify and you can easily remove it. Pour the broth into small containers and keep it in the freezer. You will have an almost fat-free broth to use anytime you need it.

To defat canned broth, try a trick I learned from Tom Ney, the director of the Food Center at *Prevention* magazine: Place an unopened can of broth in the refrigerator for several hours before using. (You can unpack the cans right into the refrigerator from the market.) When ready to use, open the can and remove the congealed fat on the top. Refrigerate or freeze in a nonmetallic container for later use. Please note that the nutrition analyses for the Chicken Broth and Vegetable Broth on pages 131 and 133 are based on unsalted commercial products.

Tamari or **soy sauce** is always called for in the low-sodium form. I prefer tamari sauce because it has a fuller flavor than soy sauce. It is also less likely to contain caramel coloring and other additives that are routinely added to most supermarket brands of soy sauce. While low-sodium soy sauce is on practically every supermarket shelf, low-sodium tamari is a bit more of a challenge to find. Some varieties contain a small amount of alcohol as a preservative, so read the label when you do find it if you want to avoid that.

Garlic and **tomato paste concentrates** both have very intense flavor. Separately, or combined, they can pick up the tenor of a recipe, especially when you're trying to cut down on fat. Each of these concentrates contains some oil to preserve freshness, but I think it's a worthwhile trade-off. You can easily substitute and use just a teaspoon or two of these unique pastes for several *tablespoons* of oil. They come in a tube which is often packed in a box (just like toothpaste!) and tomato paste concentrate is frequently found in the section with other canned tomato pastes.

Rabbit and **venison** are two of the leanest and most popular game meats available. Because of the widespread attention they've been receiving (since they're low in fat, yet high in protein, iron, and other nutrients), I included a few recipes for each. In the Resources section (page 225) you'll find listings for companies that mail-order these and other specialty items. I have found, however, that more and more local butchers are either carrying game or are happy to order it for you.

Canned beans are listed as "rinsed and drained." The rinsing is suggested for those who wish to remove excess sodium used in canning. (The USDA says there are no studies to date that confirm any significant loss of nutrients from rinsing.) You can look for the wide variety of Eden brand canned beans, which have no added salt and are very low in sodium. I recommend cooking beans from scratch. They have superior flavor, freeze beautifully for several months, and are always ready when you are.

Parmesan cheese should be freshly grated from Reggiano cheese whenever possible. Commercially packaged Parmesan and Romano cheeses are considerably higher in sodium and lack the flavor of the fresh variety.

WHAT ARE PYRAMID EQUIVALENTS?

By now you know that the Pyramid is based on a range of numbers of servings for each category of food. For instance, the recommendation is six to eleven servings of cereals and grains. That may be easier to figure out for some foods than for others. A medium baked potato is clearly one serving. A half of an English muffin is also easy to see. But when it comes to mixed dishes and recipes it's another story, and there is lots of room for confusion.

One recipe for rice pilaf may say that it serves four people. If you were to measure how much rice each person got it might be 2 cups. Another rice pilaf recipe that also serves four people might yield 1½ cups of rice per person. Does each of those recipe yields mean the same "serving" in terms of the Food Pyramid? No. A serving of rice, remember, is ½ cup; so the first recipe contributes four Pyramid servings, while the second gives three servings.

I have figured that out for you and given **Pyramid Equivalents**—for each portion—at the end of most recipes. (For some, like salad dressings, where the ingredients don't quite fit a serving, only the nutrition analysis is given. Since calcium is lost when the liquid is drained from yogurt, yield figures are not yet available. Only the nutrition analysis is given for Basic Yogurt Cream/Cheese, Creamy Orange Cheese, and Sun-dried Tomato and Garlic Dip.) That will make it faster and easier for you to know roughly where you stand and what else you can plan for that meal or eat for the rest of the day.

This is not in any way trying to box you in or turn this into a stuffy, clinical kind of diet program. So please, please, don't get caught up in the numbers. My hope is that Pyramid Equivalents will serve as an illustration that a "helping" can be more (or less) than a serving. When you keep the ideas of variety and moderation in mind you'll always come out a winner.

For the sake of brevity any bread, cereal, rice, or pasta item is a **Bread** equivalent; milk, cheese, or yogurt items are **Milk** equivalents; meat, poultry, and fish are **ounces cooked meat, poultry, or fish**, and dried beans, eggs, and nuts equivalents are given in **ounces meat alternate.**

In some cases the equivalents might actually be a tad more or less than stated, because I rounded them off to the closest familiar number, but they give you a good picture of what you're getting. In terms of the protein, that's clearly stated in ounces per portion, since the recommendation is for 5 to 7 ounces per day. That equivalent is derived from meat, poultry, fish, and game ingredients, as well as lentils, beans, and other legumes. You'll also notice how the amount of meat begins to decline in the recipes.

Several recipes showcase meats as a "center of the plate" item with 4 ounces per serving, while others have 2 ounces of meat per person. This approach uses meat as a condiment or flavoring. Smaller amounts also help you to spread the 5 to 7 ounces out over the day.

Then there are some recipes that are totally meatless, for vegetarians or those who are opting for a few meatless meals a week.

The Food Pyramid is not in any way suggesting that we eliminate meat from our menus and become vegetarians. It is asking us to look at the amount of all foods we are eating. Then it is suggesting that we eat them with a sense of "proportionality"— another way of saying moderation. As a nutritionist, I can't emphasize this point too strongly. The goal of the Pyramid, and my goal as a dietitian, is to help people maintain the best health possible by making healthy food choices. That should not require *eliminating* any food at all.

If you have physical or other health complications, these issues should be dealt with individually with the guidance of your physician and/or a registered dietitian. Ultimately pleasure, satisfaction, and good health is where we're all headed.

Enjoy the recipes.

▲▲

BEGIN WITH BREAKFAST

BAKED ORANGE FRENCH TOAST

CALIFORNIA APRICOT WAFFLES

DOUBLE-DUTY WAFFLES OR PANCAKES

TRIPLE-APPLE BRAN MUFFINS

LOW-FAT CRANBERRY MUFFINS

CINNAMON-SCENTED APRICOT BREAD

MUESLI CEREAL

WHOLE-WHEAT PEAR COUSCOUS

GINGERED FRUIT COMPOTE WITH YOGURT CREAM

PURE FRUIT MAGIC

FRESH MANGO SHAKE

▲▲

Though breakfast is enjoying brisk sales in restaurants and coffee shops, it's often the forgotten meal at home. Few people want to take the time or trouble to fix breakfast in the morning. The recipes here may change your mind. Other than the muffins or Cinnamon-Scented Apricot Bread, none take very long to prepare.

Muffins are so popular with people of all ages that I've included several recipes. You'll be amazed at how delicious they are despite the fact that they are so low in fat. I list a whole egg or an egg substitute as an ingredient because I think batter with an egg in it makes the best muffin, especially when all or most of the other fat has been left out. I use nonfat yogurt and/or a fruit purée to make up for the lost fat (see "Desserts," page 169). The muffins are far better than most totally fat-free ones. You may choose to use two egg whites instead of an egg, or you may use a frozen egg substitute. Just be aware that the muffins will be slightly rubbery and less delicate than the ones with the whole egg. The cholesterol count on a single muffin (made with the egg) still remains under 20 milligrams, which is hardly a dent in the cholesterol allotment of 300 milligrams per day.

You can put French toast back on your table with the Baked Orange French Toast recipe here. Chances are that no one will notice you haven't used butter and a frying pan to make it either. Waffles have made a big comeback, and the California Apricot Waffles, made with some whole-wheat flour, apricots, and egg white, make them more wholesome than ever.

Pure Fruit Magic and Fresh Mango Shake are two thick, rich, and fat-free ways

47

to fit in breakfast no matter how frantically you're dashing. Pour either of them into a paper cup and take it along if necessary.

Bring breakfast back into your life. It doesn't have to be a complicated or heavy meal, but it sure is a good way to begin the day.

▲▲

BAKED ORANGE FRENCH TOAST

MAKES 4 PORTIONS

Most people fry French toast in a skillet with butter, though a few restaurants serve it deep fried. But I think you'll like this moist golden French toast that leaves the extra fat behind. Use an egg substitute if you're being very vigilant. You can also assemble this the night before and keep the pan, covered with plastic wrap, in the refrigerator. Then in the morning just preheat the oven, and you're ready to roll.

1 loaf day-old wide Italian bread, cut into 1-inch slices (about 8 ounces)
1/2 cup evaporated skimmed milk
4 egg whites
2 eggs
3 tablespoons thawed frozen orange juice concentrate
1 1/2 teaspoons grated orange peel (orange part only)
1 1/2 teaspoons vanilla
1/4 teaspoon ground nutmeg

Spray a large shallow baking pan with nonstick cooking spray. Arrange the bread slices in the pan in a single layer.

In a medium bowl whisk together the remaining ingredients until blended. Pour the mixture over the bread and turn to coat.

Let stand for 30 minutes (or cover with plastic and refrigerate until ready to use); turn slices again to soak up all the egg mixture.

Preheat oven to 325° F. Bake bread for 10 minutes; turn slices over and bake for about 10 minutes longer, or until golden.

PYRAMID EQUIVALENT: 2 BREADS, 1/4 MILK, 1/2 OUNCE MEAT ALTERNATE

Nutritional Analysis per Portion

calories 263 ▲ carbohydrate 39 grams ▲ protein 14 grams ▲ fat 5 grams
sodium 455 milligrams ▲ cholesterol 108 milligrams

▲▲

CALIFORNIA APRICOT WAFFLES

MAKES 6 WAFFLES; 6 PORTIONS

Here's a chance for you to discover the reason to keep some canned apricots (or peaches, or pears) on your shelf. These yummy waffles have all the goodness of whole wheat, fruit, and buttermilk, which no one can resist. You might want to top them with some Yogurt Cream (page 65), or some of Granny's Applesauce (page 129). These waffles freeze beautifully, wrapped in an airtight bag. Reheat them in your toaster oven or toaster.

    1 cup EACH all-purpose flour and whole-wheat flour
    1 1/2 teaspoons baking powder
    1/2 teaspoon baking soda
    1/4 teaspoon salt, optional
    2 cups low-fat (1%) buttermilk
    2 egg whites
    1 egg
    1 tablespoon EACH canola oil and vanilla extract
    1 tablespoon packed brown sugar
    1 16-ounce can apricot halves, in light syrup, well drained and diced (re-
        serve juice for another use)

Preheat waffle iron according to manufacturer's instructions. Spray with nonstick cooking spray (unless iron has a nonstick surface).

In a large bowl whisk together the flours, baking powder, baking soda, and salt, if using; set aside.

In a medium bowl whisk together the remaining ingredients until frothy and sugar is dissolved; stir into dry ingredients until just moistened. Pour about ¾ cup* of the batter onto preheated iron; cook according to manufacturer's instructions. (Because of the added fruit, waffle may need an extra minute to cook.) Serve immediately.

* Waffle irons come in various sizes and shapes; follow the instructions for your unit.

PYRAMID EQUIVALENT: 2 BREADS, ⅓ FRUIT, ⅓ MILK

Nutritional Analysis per Portion

calories 289 ▲ carbohydrate 50 grams ▲ protein 10 grams ▲ fat 5 grams
sodium 345 milligrams ▲ cholesterol 40 milligrams

▲▲▲

DOUBLE-DUTY WAFFLES OR PANCAKES

MAKES FOUR WAFFLES OR
EIGHT 4-IN. PANCAKES; 4 PORTIONS

This versatile recipe can be used on the waffle iron or griddle. I sometimes add some corn kernels or currants or dried apples to give them a new look. Because they're made with egg whites, they tend to brown less evenly than waffles made with whole eggs. You can also double this recipe to make a double batch. They freeze beautifully.

½ cup EACH all-purpose flour and whole-wheat flour
¾ teaspoon baking powder
½ teaspoon baking soda
1 cup lowfat (1.5%) buttermilk
2 egg whites
2 tablespoons maple syrup
2 teaspoons vegetable oil

Preheat waffle iron, if you're using one, according to manufacturer's instructions. Spray with nonstick cooking spray (unless iron has a nonstick surface).

In a large bowl whisk together the flours, baking powder, and baking soda; set aside.

In a medium bowl whisk together the remaining ingredients until frothy; stir into dry ingredients until just moistened.

For Waffles: Pour about ½ cup* of the batter onto preheated iron; cook according to manufacturer's instructions. Serve immediately.

For Pancakes: Spray a large skillet with nonstick cooking spray and heat over medium-high heat. Pour about ¼ cup batter into skillet for each pancake. Cook for about 3 minutes or until bubbles appear and the undersides are lightly browned. Turn the cakes over and cook 1 to 2 minutes longer.

* Waffle irons come in various sizes and shapes; follow the instructions for your unit.

PYRAMID EQUIVALENT: 1¼ BREADS, ¼ MILK

Nutritional Analysis per Portion

calories 200 ▲ carbohydrate 33 grams ▲ protein 8 grams ▲ fat 4 grams
sodium 354 milligrams ▲ cholesterol 3 milligrams

▲▲▲

TRIPLE-APPLE BRAN MUFFINS

MAKES 12 MUFFINS; 12 PORTIONS

Each of these moist, high-fiber muffins is very low in fat, and low in cholesterol. Everyone will enjoy them. Apple juice, applesauce, and pieces of fresh apple replace much of the fat with lots of flavor. They freeze well, so you can always have some on hand.

1 cup bran cereal, crushed

1 5$\frac{1}{2}$-ounce can unsweetened apple juice

1$\frac{3}{4}$ cups all-purpose flour

1 tablespoon baking powder

2 teaspoons ground cinnamon

$\frac{1}{2}$ teaspoon salt

$\frac{3}{4}$ cup unsweetened applesauce

1 egg

2 tablespoons vegetable oil

$\frac{1}{4}$ cup EACH granulated sugar and packed dark brown sugar

$\frac{1}{2}$ cup fresh chopped apple

Preheat oven to 375° F. Spray a 12-cup muffin tin with nonstick cooking spray; set aside.

In a small bowl combine cereal and apple juice; let stand until cereal is softened, about 5 minutes.

Meanwhile in a large bowl whisk together flour, baking powder, cinnamon, and salt; set aside.

In a medium bowl whisk together applesauce, egg, vegetable oil, and sugars.

Make a well in the center of the flour mixture. Pour in bran mixture, applesauce mixture, and stir until just combined; fold in apples. Spoon batter into prepared muffin tin. Bake 20 to 25 minutes, or until a tester inserted in center comes out clean.

Cool muffins in pan on a wire rack for 3 minutes. Turn onto rack to finish cooling. Serve warm or completely cooled.

PYRAMID EQUIVALENT: $\frac{3}{4}$ BREAD, $\frac{1}{4}$ FRUIT

Nutritional Analysis per Portion

calories 163 ▲ carbohydrate 32 grams ▲ protein 3 grams ▲ fat 3 grams
sodium 268 milligrams ▲ cholesterol 18 milligrams

▲▲▲

LOW-FAT CRANBERRY MUFFINS

MAKES 12 MUFFINS; 12 PORTIONS

Even when you use a whole egg in this recipe, the amount of fat per muffin is low, and the cholesterol is less than 20 milligrams each.

Cranberries make a tart addition to this not-too-sweet treat, which needn't be limited to breakfast. You can also use frozen or fresh blueberries if you like. Neither of the berries have to be thawed if they are frozen. For variety I sometimes whirl 1 cup of rolled oats in a blender and substitute it for the whole-wheat flour.

1¼ cups cake flour
¾ cup whole-wheat flour
1½ teaspoons EACH baking powder and baking soda
½ teaspoon EACH ground cinnamon and ground cloves
¼ teaspoon salt
¾ cup nonfat plain yogurt
½ cup unsweetened applesauce
⅓ cup packed brown sugar
1 egg or 2 egg whites or ¼ cup frozen egg substitute, thawed
1½ cups fresh cranberries

Preheat oven to 375° F. Spray 12 muffin cups with nonstick cooking spray; set aside.

In a medium bowl whisk together the flours, baking powder, baking soda, cinnamon, cloves, and salt; set aside.

In another medium bowl whisk together the remaining ingredients, except the cranberries, breaking up the brown sugar.

Make a well in the center of the flour mixture. Pour in applesauce mixture, and stir until just combined (do not overmix); fold in cranberries. Spoon batter into prepared muffin tin. Bake 20 to 25 minutes, or until a tester inserted in center comes out clean.

Cool muffins in pan on a wire rack for 3 minutes. Turn onto rack to finish cooling. Serve warm or completely cooled.

PYRAMID EQUIVALENT: 1 BREAD, ¼ FRUIT

Nutritional Analysis per Portion

calories 117 ▲ carbohydrate 24 grams ▲ protein 3 grams ▲ fat 1 gram
sodium 282 milligrams ▲ cholesterol 18 milligrams

▲▲▲

CINNAMON-SCENTED APRICOT BREAD

MAKES 1 LOAF; 10 PORTIONS

This low-fat loaf freezes as well as any rich, buttery cousin. Dried apricots give it a nice tart edge while the cinnamon keeps it mellow. Use the Apricot Purée (page 177) or apricot baby food instead of the applesauce if you like.

½ cup plus 2 teaspoons sugar
1¾ teaspoons ground cinnamon
1½ cups all-purpose flour
½ cup whole-wheat flour
1¼ teaspoons baking powder
1 teaspoon baking soda
½ teaspoon salt
1¼ cups unsweetened applesauce
2 tablespoons vegetable oil
2 egg whites, at room temperature
1 egg
½ cup chopped dried apricots
2 teaspoons grated orange peel (orange part only)

54

Preheat oven to 350° F. Spray a 9 × 5-inch loaf pan with nonstick cooking spray; set aside.

In a small bowl combine the 2 teaspoons of sugar and ¼ teaspoon of the cinnamon; set aside.

In a large bowl whisk together the flours, ½ cup sugar, baking powder, baking soda, remaining cinnamon, and salt; set aside.

In a medium bowl whisk together the applesauce, oil, egg whites, and egg until blended; whisk in apricots and orange peel. Make a well in the center of the flour mixture. Pour in applesauce mixture, and stir until just combined. Spoon batter into prepared pan. Sprinkle reserved sugar/cinnamon evenly over the top of batter.

Bake 45 to 50 minutes, or until a tester inserted in center comes out clean. Cool in pan on a wire rack for 10 minutes. Turn onto rack to finish cooling. Serve warm or completely cooled.

PYRAMID EQUIVALENT:
1 BREAD, ¼ FRUIT

Nutritional Analysis per Portion

calories 196 ▲ carbohydrate 38 grams ▲ protein 4 grams ▲ fat 4 grams
sodium 316 milligrams ▲ cholesterol 21 milligrams

▲▲▲

MUESLI CEREAL

MAKES 4 PORTIONS

You get the royal treatment when you order this health-minded cereal at the sophisticated Rihga Royal Hotel in New York City. It's easy to make at home, and making it the night before means it's ready and waiting when you are.

1 1/3 cups old-fashioned uncooked rolled oats
1/3 cup toasted unsweetened wheat germ
1/4 cup EACH dark and light raisins
1 tablespoon EACH orange marmalade and honey
1/2 teaspoon ground cinnamon
3 cups low-fat (1%) milk
2 tablespoons shelled sunflower seeds
Chopped nuts, to taste (optional; may include walnuts, pecans, almonds, etc.)

In a large mixing bowl combine all ingredients except sunflower seeds. Cover and refrigerate overnight.

To serve, stir cereal mixture, and ladle into serving bowl. Sprinkle with seeds and nuts if desired.

PYRAMID EQUIVALENT (NOT INCLUDING CHOPPED NUTS):
1 1/2 BREADS, 1/2 FRUIT, 3/4 MILK

Nutritional Analysis per Portion

calories 326 ▲ carbohydrate 57 grams ▲ protein 15 grams ▲ fat 7 grams
sodium 96 milligrams ▲ cholesterol 7 milligrams

▲▲▲

WHOLE-WHEAT PEAR COUSCOUS

MAKES 4 PORTIONS

Pear nectar and cardamom round out the flavors in this simple high-fiber breakfast. You won't need any extra sugar for this naturally sweet cereal either. A splash of low-fat milk, or a dollop of Yogurt Cream (page 65) will finish it off nicely.

1½ cups (one 12-ounce can) pear nectar
1½ cups water
½ cup snipped pitted prunes
1⅓ cups quick-cooking whole-wheat couscous
¼ teaspoon ground cardamom or cinnamon

In a medium saucepan bring the nectar and water to a boil. Add the remaining ingredients. Cover, reduce heat to low, and cook for 5 minutes.

PYRAMID EQUIVALENT: 1¾ BREADS, 1 FRUIT

Nutritional Analysis per Portion

calories 335 ▲ carbohydrate 75 grams ▲ protein 8 grams ▲ fat 1 gram
sodium 11 milligrams ▲ cholesterol 0 milligrams

▲▲

GINGERED FRUIT COMPOTE WITH YOGURT CREAM

MAKES 4 PORTIONS

Prunes pack a nutritious punch: they're loaded with fiber, iron, vitamin A, and potassium. This easy recipe lets you serve them in a way that will have people begging for seconds.

1 cup pitted prunes (about 6 ounces)
1 large Granny Smith apple, peeled and cut into 1-inch cubes
¾ cup orange juice
¼ cup water
2 teaspoons grated fresh gingerroot
1 teaspoon grated orange peel (orange part only)
1 cup (one 11-ounce can) mandarin orange segments, drained
Yogurt Cream (page 65), optional

In a medium saucepan combine all the ingredients, except the orange sections and Yogurt Cream. Bring to a boil. Reduce heat to medium-low, cover, and cook for 5 minutes, or until apples are tender. Cover and chill until ready to use. Just before serving, stir in the orange sections. Spoon into dessert dishes. Place 2 tablespoons of Yogurt Cream on each portion, if desired.

PYRAMID EQUIVALENT: 1 FRUIT

Nutritional Analysis per Portion

calories 192 ▲ carbohydrate 50 grams ▲ protein 2 grams ▲ fat 0 grams
sodium 7 milligrams ▲ cholesterol 0 milligrams

▲▲

PURE FRUIT MAGIC

MAKES 2 PORTIONS

It's magic that this drink tastes so rich without any milk or other fillers to boost it up. Try any of your favorite berries, and toss in some melon, peaches, or pears. Keep the banana, however; it's what gives this shake its underlying smoothness.

Now that I own a Cuisinart Quick Prep hand blender (immersion blender), I make these drinks all the time, not just for breakfast.

1 1/2 cups blueberries
1 small banana, cut in three pieces
1/2 cup unsweetened pineapple juice
1/2 teaspoon vanilla, optional
4 ice cubes

In a blender combine all the ingredients until thick and smooth.

▲▲▲

FRESH MANGO SHAKE

MAKES I PORTION

I am totally mad about mangoes. Once you know which ones to look for, and how to slice them, it's no longer a battle of the knife. Look for Mexican mangoes, which tend to be less "hairy" and stringy than the Haitian ones. The real trick to freeing the fruit from the pit is to use a thin, sharp vegetable knife. Cut through to the pit in about a one-quarter section; slide the knife under the flesh and ease the wedge off the pit. Then slide the knife between the skin and the fruit to remove the peel.

Mangoes are a good source of fiber, and an outstanding source of beta carotene and vitamin A.

I small mango (about 8 ounces), quartered, pitted, and peeled
¾ cup nonfat plain yogurt
⅓ cup orange juice
2 ice cubes

In a blender combine all the ingredients until thick and smooth.

▲▲▲▲▲▲▲▲▲▲▲▲▲▲▲▲▲▲▲▲▲▲▲▲▲▲▲▲▲▲▲▲▲▲▲▲▲▲

APPETIZERS, SOUPS, AND BREADS

BASIC YOGURT CREAM/CHEESE

CREAMY ORANGE CHEESE

YOGURT CHEESE VARIATIONS

SUN-DRIED TOMATO AND GARLIC DIP

GREEK GARLIC-POTATO DIP

ITALIAN GARLIC TOASTS

HERBED WHITE BEAN DIP

SEASONED ITALIAN TOMATOES

NICK'S PITA CHIPS

PIZZA BITES

SMOKY SPLIT PEA SOUP

SWISS CHARD SOUP

SILKY SWEET POTATO AND APPLE BISQUE

CHILLED MANGO AND MELON SOUP

HANDS-OFF WHOLE-WHEAT CORNMEAL BREAD

YOGURT-CHIVE BATTER BREAD WITH POPPY SEEDS

SAVORY PEPPERED CORN MUFFINS

FOCACCIA WITH ONIONS, ROSEMARY, AND FETA CHEESE

STEAMED CHINESE BUNS

▲▲▲

I have to admit that for years I rarely served appetizers. I did put out the ubiquitous platter of fresh vegetables and a dip for company, but overall this category is a challenging one for me. Even in restaurants, I generally don't order an appetizer. For the most part, the foods we tend to serve as hors d'oeuvres are loaded with fat. Assorted nuts, platters of rich cheeses, pâtés, sour cream–based dips, and fried this-and-that are just not my idea of how to begin a meal.

Hospitality and hungry guests, however, do mandate premeal tidbits that are more than raw or steamed vegetables. So over the last few years I have tried to come up with some appetizer recipes that are light yet satisfying. Coincidentally they fit right in with the Pyramid guidelines. These recipes are low in fat or fat-free, some are high in fiber, and all are packed with flavor, just the right combination to whet the appetite for the meal to come.

I included some bread recipes in this section for you to ponder before you get too far along in menu planning. The yeast bread recipes take several hours to make, so here's your advance notice. The Focaccia, however, can be made with frozen pizza dough, which saves you a lot of time and energy.

Since just about everybody loves cheese and creamy dips, I am giving you directions on how to make yogurt cheese. I was first introduced to this several years ago by a dietitian friend of mine, Marlene Lauzze, in Syracuse, New York. Both she and her husband Jerry are fat-avoiding fanatics, so I was puzzled when they served me a rich, creamy herb-peppered cheese. It turned out that what I was eating was really low-fat yogurt that had been drained overnight in the refrigerator. I've been captivated ever since.

I do hope you'll try some of the other appetizer recipes. Greek Garlic-Potato Dip and Herbed White Bean Dip get you well on your way to filling your quota for complex carbohydrates for the day. Seasoned Italian Tomatoes is about the best way I know to serve ripe summer tomatoes.

Soups have always been a favorite category among comfort foods, yet they are often filled with butter, cream, and sometimes eggs to thicken and enrich them. Smoky Split Pea Soup, however, is thick and satisfying without a drop of fat or oil added. Silky Sweet Potato and Apple Bisque is as rich as a soup can get, and potatoes are the reason why.

Do try some of the recipes for breads. Hands-off Whole-Wheat Cornmeal Bread is made in a bread machine (conventional instructions are also provided), so there's practically no effort at all. I am especially fond of Savory Peppered Corn Muffins. They are studded with cooked dried peas, very low in fat, and a snap to make.

YOGURT CREAM/CHEESE PRIMER

To me, one of the neatest ways to enjoy yogurt—especially nonfat yogurt—is to drain it and use it as a rich sauce or a dip, or as a cheese. This "cheese" can be used as is, blended with other flavorings, or used as a sumptuous ingredient in other dishes. The best part is there's absolutely no fat, though the taste and texture may tell you otherwise.

Here's the way to make it and some tips for other uses:

Place some cheesecloth or a paper towel in a large strainer or colander, and set this over a bowl. Spoon the yogurt into the strainer. Place in the refrigerator overnight or for a few hours. The longer it sits the thicker and creamier it gets. If you want to use the yogurt for a sauce, an hour or two should do it. For cheese, six to twenty-four hours of draining is needed.

You can also buy a yogurt cheese funnel (see Really Creamy, in Resources, page 225). This handy device incorporates a special micro-size mesh that encourages quick drainage. Check the housewares area of most department stores or ask at your local health food store. The package includes filters, a cone, and recipes for several variations.

I suggest you test your yogurt before you make the first batch. Most yogurts can be drained, but a few brands cannot because they contain certain gelatins or stabilizers. (Gelatin holds the whey in the yogurt so that it will not separate.)

Plain, vanilla, French vanilla, lemon, or coffee flavors work best; the fruit varieties work well. Check first by placing a heaping tablespoon of yogurt in a small dish. Make a depression in the center and wait about ten minutes. If some liquid starts to accumulate, you should be able to go on with the process. And if there is already some liquid at the top of the container when you open it, you don't need to test it; it has begun to drain on its own. This liquid that drains off is whey, the watery portion of milk that is traditionally separated from the milk in cheese making.

Yogurt cheese is quick and easy to make at home. Depending on how long you let it drain, one quart of yogurt will yield 1½ to 2 cups of cheese. Always store the final product in a covered container in the refrigerator; it should last for one to two weeks.

Try different brands for different flavor characteristics. You will quickly learn to know from just one spoonful how the final yogurt sauce or cheese will taste. Some are quite tangy, while others are milder or creamier (even though they are nonfat). This difference depends on the type of yogurt culture used, the fermentation process, and/or the stabilizers or additives—if any—that are used by the manufacturers. For instance, I often use Dannon for a dessert sauce, because it starts out with a softer flavor than, say, Axelrod, which has a traditional tart yogurt taste. So Axelrod will be right in a cheese where I will be adding herbs. Play around and experiment. Chances are you already have a preference that is based on the element of tartness.

▲▲

BASIC YOGURT CREAM/CHEESE

MAKES 1½ TO 2 CUPS

Use this recipe as the base for both sweet and savory dishes. Please see the Yogurt Cream/Cheese Primer (page 64) for a complete explanation of this wondrous use of yogurt and pages 67–68 for other suggestions.

1 quart nonfat plain yogurt

Place a double layer of cheesecloth, a paper towel, or a paper coffee filter in a large strainer or colander and set this over a bowl.* Place in the refrigerator for 1 to 3 hours for soft cheese (cream) or dip or overnight to make a fuller, richer cheese.

* Yogurt cheese filters can be purchased in department stores, health food stores, or by mail. See page 225 for ordering information.

Nutritional Analysis per Cup

calories 160 ▲ carbohydrate 17 grams ▲ protein 18 grams ▲ fat 0 grams
sodium 160 milligrams ▲ cholesterol 0 milligrams

▲▲

CREAMY ORANGE CHEESE

MAKES ABOUT 1 ½ CUPS

What a great topping this makes for bagels. No one will guess it's totally fat-free. Use a light, mild honey for a delicate flavor balance.

    1 quart nonfat plain yogurt
    2 teaspoons honey
    2 teaspoons thawed frozen orange juice concentrate
    ½ teaspoon grated orange peel (orange part only)

Drain yogurt according to directions above, leaving it in the refrigerator overnight.

   In a medium bowl combine yogurt with remaining ingredients until blended. Cover and keep in refrigerator until ready to serve.

▲▲▲

YOGURT CHEESE VARIATIONS

Play around with the consistency and the flavor to make your own variations. You might want a light orange sauce for pancakes, waffles, or French toast instead of butter. Let the yogurt drain for just about an hour and stir in some orange juice and/ or grated orange peel. On the other hand, maybe you're looking for some new hors d'oeuvre or canapé ideas. This is the time to drain the yogurt overnight and add some spices, as suggested for spicy and savory uses, on the next page.

For a touch of sweetness:

▲ Add a teaspoon or two of honey, maple syrup, or light molasses to taste.

▲ Stir in thawed frozen orange, apple, or other fruit juice concentrate to taste.

▲ Blend in a bit of pure fruit preserves.

▲ Mix in a teaspoon or two of confectioners' sugar and grated orange or lemon peel; or use a pinch of ground cinnamon, nutmeg, cardamom, or ginger instead of the grated peel.

▲ Purée leftover or slightly overripe fruits like bananas, grapes, berries, peaches, or plums, and fold into the yogurt.

For spicy and savory uses:

▲ Add some finely minced shallots, garlic, onion, or jalapeño pepper.

▲ Stir in some Mexican salsa and serve with vegetables.

▲ Add fresh or dried herbs like basil, cilantro, or tarragon, with a bit of cracked pepper, and spread on crackers or thinly sliced whole-grain breads.

▲ Make a mustard sauce for fish, chicken, or vegetables by stirring in a teaspoon of Dijon mustard, some lemon juice to taste, and maybe even some fresh herbs like dill, chives, or chervil.

▲▲▲

SUN-DRIED TOMATO AND GARLIC DIP

MAKES 6 PORTIONS

Most supermarkets and specialty stores now carry concentrated tomato and garlic pastes packed in tubes. They are strongly flavored and pack the true essence of each vegetable. If you are unable to find them, use regular tomato paste or roasted garlic* as stand-ins.

    1 quart low-fat or nonfat plain yogurt
    1 tablespoon plus 1 teaspoon sun-dried tomato paste from tube
    1 teaspoon garlic paste from tube or 2 to 3 garlic cloves, minced
    1 teaspoon finely minced basil, optional
    ⅛ teaspoon freshly ground black pepper, or to taste
    Basil leaves to garnish, optional

Drain the yogurt according to directions on page 66, leaving it in the refrigerator for 4 to 6 hours, or until creamy.

In a medium bowl combine the yogurt with remaining ingredients, except whole basil leaves, until blended. Cover and refrigerate until ready to serve. Garnish with basil leaves, if desired.

* To roast garlic: Preheat oven to 350° F. Lightly rub 6 large unpeeled garlic cloves with water and roast them in a small baking dish for about 30 minutes, or until soft and tender. Squeeze each clove to extract purée.

Nutritional Analysis per Portion (low-fat yogurt)

calories 70 ▲ carbohydrate 4 grams ▲ protein 7 grams ▲ fat 2 grams
sodium 77 milligrams ▲ cholesterol 4 milligrams

▲▲

GREEK GARLIC-POTATO DIP

MAKES 8 PORTIONS

Skordalia, the Greek dip/sauce, has numerous variations, but garlic is its essential ingredient (*skorda* is the Greek word for garlic). It is often made with lima beans, bread, or potato. This version uses the good old American spud; it is especially nice made with Yukon Gold potatoes. Their waxy, almost buttery consistency makes up for the reduced amount of oil used here. Serve the dip with raw vegetables or Nick's Pita Chips (page 73).

4 medium potatoes, cooked, peeled, and cubed (about 1 1/4 pounds)
5 large garlic cloves, pressed
1 cup nonfat plain yogurt
3 tablespoons fresh lemon juice
2 tablespoons extra-virgin olive oil
1 teaspoon salt
Dash ground red pepper
1/3 cup chopped Italian (flat-leaf) parsley

While the potatoes are still warm, in a large bowl, using an electric mixer on medium speed, beat potatoes until smooth and almost lump-free. Add the remaining ingredients, except the parsley, and beat until thoroughly combined.

Scrape the mixture into a medium bowl, and stir in the parsley. Cover and refrigerate for several hours to let the flavors blend. Bring almost to room temperature before serving.

PYRAMID EQUIVALENT: ½ VEGETABLE

Nutritional Analysis per Portion

calories 106 ▲ carbohydrate 16 grams ▲ protein 3 grams ▲ fat 4 grams
sodium 300 milligrams ▲ cholesterol 1 milligram

▲▲▲

ITALIAN GARLIC TOASTS

(CROSTINI)

MAKES 8 PORTIONS

Crostini is the Italian word for small toasts, or croutons. They are usually brushed with a liberal amount of olive oil before toasting, but the crunchy tidbits here are without oil. You can top *crostini* with an herbed cheese mixture or an herbed tomato mixture such as the one on page 72.

    1 loaf baguette-style bread (about 8 ounces) bias-sliced into ½-inch pieces
        (about 32)
    3 large garlic cloves, halved

Preheat oven to 350° F.

Place the bread slices on a large baking sheet. Bake for about 10 minutes, or until lightly browned and crusty.

70

When the bread slices are just cool enough to handle, rub both sides lightly with raw garlic halves (the garlic should almost melt into the toast).

Let cool and store in an airtight container for up to a week.

PYRAMID EQUIVALENT (ABOUT 4 TOASTS): I BREAD

Nutritional Analysis per Portion

calories 79 ▲ carbohydrate 15 grams ▲ protein 3 grams ▲ fat I gram
sodium 166 milligrams ▲ cholesterol 0 milligrams

▲▲

HERBED WHITE BEAN DIP

MAKES 4 PORTIONS

Here's another fat-free spread you can serve with Nick's Pita Chips (page 73), and to top Italian Garlic Toasts (opposite). It takes less than a minute to make, and when I'm really pressed for time I tear open a bag of Guiltless Gourmet no-oil tortilla chips, which are baked—not fried—to go with it.

2 cups cooked white beans or canned beans, rinsed and drained
$1/2$ teaspoon EACH dried marjoram, basil, and thyme, crumbled
I tablespoon fresh lemon juice
I teaspoon capers plus 2 teaspoons of the liquid
$1/4$ teaspoon ground white pepper

In the workbowl of a food processor pulse the beans once or twice, until slightly mashed. Add the remaining ingredients, and pulse two or three more times or until just combined. Adjust seasonings if necessary.

PYRAMID EQUIVALENT: 1 VEGETABLE, OR 1 OUNCE MEAT ALTERNATE

Nutritional Analysis per Portion

calories 127 ▴ carbohydrate 23 grams ▴ protein 9 grams ▴ fat 0 grams
sodium 44 milligrams ▴ cholesterol 0 milligrams

▲▲

SEASONED ITALIAN TOMATOES

MAKES 6 PORTIONS

Use this lively mixture as a topping for Italian Garlic Toasts (page 70), on top of diagonal slices of zucchini or yellow squash, or to fill leaves of fresh Belgian endive. Any way you choose, it's an elegant and attractive hors d'oeuvre. Though I prefer plum tomatoes, use any tomatoes that are fully ripe and flavorful.

2 cups plum tomatoes, seeded and cut into 1/4-inch dice (about 1 1/4 pounds)
1/4 cup finely chopped red onion
1/4 cup EACH chopped fresh parsley and basil leaves
2 tablespoons chopped oil-cured Italian olives
2 tablespoons balsamic vinegar, or to taste
Salt and freshly ground black pepper, to taste

In a medium bowl combine all the ingredients. Let stand for 30 minutes at room temperature, or cover and refrigerate until ready to serve. Bring back to room temperature. Adjust seasonings to taste.

PYRAMID EQUIVALENT: 1/2 VEGETABLE

Nutritional Analysis per Portion

calories 34 ▴ carbohydrate 6 grams ▴ protein 1 gram ▴ fat 1 gram
sodium 108 milligrams ▴ cholesterol 0 milligrams

▲▲▲

NICK'S PITA CHIPS

MAKES 8 PORTIONS (ABOUT 32 CHIPS)

Serve these crisp and practically fat-free pita toasts with the Sun-dried Tomato and Garlic Dip (page 68). Nick Danielides, a good friend and great cook, livens up these easy snacks with a touch of sesame oil and a sprinkling of sesame seeds. His two young boys love them so much they clamor to have a few as a bedtime snack.

   1 egg white
   1/2 teaspoon sesame oil
   8 6-inch pita breads (about 2 ounces each), cut in quarters
   2 teaspoons sesame seeds

Preheat oven to 350° F.

In a small bowl whisk together the egg white and oil. Place pita quarters on a nonstick baking sheet. Lightly brush both sides with egg mixture; sprinkle seeds evenly over bread.

Bake for about 10 minutes, or until golden brown. Turn chips over and bake about 5 minutes longer.

PYRAMID EQUIVALENT: 2 BREADS

Nutritional Analysis per Portion

calories 174 ▲ carbohydrate 34 grams ▲ protein 6 grams ▲ fat 1 gram
sodium 329 milligrams ▲ cholesterol 0 milligrams

▲▲▲

PIZZA BITES

MAKES 60 BITES; 15 PORTIONS

Carol Gelles, author of *Wholesome Harvest*, introduced me to these tasty morsels of baked, seasoned pizza dough. My version uses some whole-wheat flour and a touch of honey. Pizza dough is quite easy to make by hand, and if you have a bread machine it's almost effortless.

 2¹/₂ cups all-purpose flour
 ¹/₂ cup whole-wheat flour
 1 package quick-rise yeast
 ³/₄ teaspoon salt
 1 cup very warm water (about 130° F)
 2 tablespoons olive oil
 1¹/₂ teaspoons honey
 4 large garlic cloves, minced fine, or pressed
 1 egg white, lightly beaten, optional

Spray a large baking sheet with nonstick cooking spray; set aside.

In a large bowl combine 1 cup of the all-purpose flour, the whole-wheat flour, yeast, and salt. Stir in the water, olive oil, honey, and garlic. Stir in enough of the remaining flour to make a soft dough.

On a lightly floured surface knead dough for about 5 minutes, or until it is smooth and elastic. Cover with plastic wrap, and let rest for 10 minutes.

Punch the dough down and pinch off small pieces; roll into small balls about 1 inch in diameter. Place on prepared pan, about 1 inch apart. Cover lightly with plastic wrap and let stand for 10 minutes.

Meanwhile, preheat oven to 425° F. Brush each of the bites with some egg white, if desired. Bake for 15 minutes, or until golden. Cool on a wire rack.

Place ingredients in bread pan according to manufacturer's instructions. Select DOUGH setting. Remove dough from pan. Pinch off 1-inch pieces of dough, and proceed as directed above.

Note: This recipe also makes one 14-inch thick pizza crust, 2 12-inch thin pizza crusts, or 24 breadsticks.

PYRAMID EQUIVALENT (PER 4 BITES): 1 BREAD

Nutritional Analysis per Portion

calories 112 ▲ carbohydrate 20 grams ▲ protein 3 grams ▲ fat 2 grams
sodium 115 milligrams ▲ cholesterol 0 milligrams

▲▲▲

SMOKY SPLIT PEA SOUP

MAKES 6 APPETIZER PORTIONS
OR 4 MAIN COURSE PORTIONS

You won't find any fat in this spicy, fiber-filled soup. It's so easy to make that by the time you toss a salad and set the table, it's practically ready to serve. Dried chili peppers can be found in spice shops and gourmet specialty stores. The combination of the peppers along with the natural hickory seasoning (liquid smoke—check the supermarket spice section or health food stores for this item), gives the soup a rich flavor without calling for a ham bone. Now you can make this soup for vegetarians too. A dollop of yogurt in the center of each serving will cool the fire of the peppers.

1 pound split peas, sorted and rinsed
6 cups water
4 EACH whole cloves and black peppercorns
2 bay leaves
1 dried chili, about 1 inch across and 2 inches long*
1 3-inch cinnamon stick
2 teaspoons natural hickory seasoning (liquid smoke)
1 1/2 teaspoons salt
Chopped cilantro for garnish, optional

In a large saucepan or Dutch oven, combine all the ingredients except the salt.

Cover and bring to a boil over high heat. Reduce heat and simmer, partially covered, for about 40 minutes, or until the peas are soft. Using a slotted spoon, remove cloves, peppercorns, bay leaves, chili, and cinnamon stick.

In the workbowl of a food processor, in one or two batches (depending on the size of your processor), purée until the soup is smooth. Return the soup to the pan, add the salt, and cook for about 3 minutes, or until heated through. Ladle soup into bowls and garnish with chopped cilantro, if desired.

* If chilies are large, break into smaller pieces. *Wear plastic gloves.* Even dried, chilies require careful handling.

PYRAMID EQUIVALENT: 2 VEGETABLES (OR 2 OUNCES MEAT ALTERNATE)
AS AN APPETIZER, 3 VEGETABLES
(OR 3 OUNCES MEAT ALTERNATE) AS A MAIN COURSE

Nutritional Analysis per Portion (main course)

calories 395 ▲ carbohydrate 70 grams ▲ protein 28 grams ▲ fat 2 grams
sodium 840 milligrams ▲ cholesterol 0 milligrams

Nutritional Analysis per Portion (appetizer)

calories 263 ▲ carbohydrate 47 grams ▲ protein 19 grams ▲ fat 1 gram
sodium 561 milligrams ▲ cholesterol 0 milligrams

▲▲

SWISS CHARD SOUP

MAKES 6 PORTIONS

Felipé Rojas-Lombardi was one of the most creative and talented cooks of our time and a special acquaintance of mine. If you're a fan of soups and don't own a copy of Felipé's book *Soup, Beautiful Soup*, run out and get one: it's a treasure.

This recipe, adapted from that book, has special appeal to the nutritionist part of me because Swiss chard is loaded with vitamin A (beta carotene), potassium, and a bit of iron and calcium. Chef Lombardi liked to stir in some crème fraîche or heavy cream when reheating, but I omitted that here.

16–18 cups Swiss chard, thoroughly washed and drained (about 2 pounds)
2 tablespoons olive oil
2 large garlic cloves, minced
1 or 2 jalapeño peppers, seeded and chopped fine
2 cups finely chopped celery (about 4 stalks)
1 teaspoon ground cumin
1/8 teaspoon EACH ground cloves and ground nutmeg
2 cups finely chopped onion
1 teaspoon salt
1 cup cooked chick-peas, or canned chick-peas, rinsed and drained
5 cups water or defatted low-sodium chicken stock

Take 6 to 8 of the widest and freshest chard stems and cut into julienne strips. Place them in a bowl of chilled water; set aside. Chop the rest of the Swiss chard, both the leaves and stems; set aside.

In a large saucepan heat the oil; add the garlic, pepper, celery, cumin, cloves, and nutmeg. Cook over medium heat, stirring occasionally, for about 3 minutes, or until the celery is soft. Stir in the onion and salt, and cook for another 5 minutes, or until the onion is translucent. Add the chick-peas and Swiss chard, and cook for 8 to 10 minutes, or until the Swiss chard is wilted. Add the water or stock, cover, and bring to a boil. Reduce heat and simmer for 10 minutes. Remove from heat and cool slightly.

In the workbowl of a food processor, in one or two batches (depending on the size of your processor), process until the soup is smooth.

Return the soup to the pot, adjust seasonings, and cook for about 5 minutes, or until heated through. Meanwhile, drain reserved Swiss chard stems and pat dry with a paper towel. Serve the soup garnished with the julienned chard.

PYRAMID EQUIVALENT: 4 1/2 VEGETABLES

Nutritional Analysis per Portion

calories 145 ▲ carbohydrate 20 grams ▲ protein 6 grams ▲ fat 6 grams
sodium 728 milligrams ▲ cholesterol 0 milligrams

▲▲

SILKY SWEET POTATO AND APPLE BISQUE

MAKES 6 PORTIONS

There's just a tad of oil in this rich soup that's full of beta carotene, fiber, and good taste. The recipe comes from Pat Mason, a food writer friend of mine who lives in Maine; it had been passed on to her from three other people. Once you try it you'll know it's worth the pass-along.

1 tablespoon canola oil
2 cups chopped onion
2 pounds sweet potatoes, peeled and cut into 1-inch cubes
2 Granny Smith apples, cored, peeled, cut into 1-inch cubes (about 12 ounces)
3 cups chicken or vegetable broth (see page 40)
3/4 cup apple juice
1 teaspoon EACH dried thyme and dried basil, crushed
1/4 teaspoon freshly ground black pepper

78

In a large saucepan heat the oil over medium-high heat. Add the onion and cook for about 3 minutes, stirring occasionally, until tender. Add remaining ingredients, cover partially, and bring to a boil.

Reduce heat and simmer for about 15 minutes, or until the potatoes are tender. Cool slightly.

In the workbowl of a food processor, purée soup in several batches (depending on the size of your processor) until smooth.

Return the soup to the pan, and heat until warmed through.

PYRAMID EQUIVALENT: 1/2 FRUIT, 1 1/2 VEGETABLES

Nutritional Analysis per Portion

calories 214 ▲ carbohydrate 43 grams ▲ protein 4 grams ▲ fat 4 grams
sodium 44 milligrams ▲ cholesterol 0 milligrams

▲▲▲

CHILLED MANGO AND MELON SOUP

MAKES 4 PORTIONS

Many fruit soups require cooking to bring out the full flavor of the fruit—not this one. Instead, the ingredients are whirled together in a food processor, then the flavors develop while chilling in the refrigerator. Mangoes and melons are in the market almost all year long as more produce is shipped in from other countries. That means you have more time to enjoy this luscious soup.

Juice of 2 large limes and 8 thin strips of peel from 1 lime, green part only,
     for garnish
3 cups cubed cantaloupe or honeydew melon
1 large ripe mango, peeled, pitted, and cubed
3/4 cup orange juice

79

In the workbowl of a food processor, purée all ingredients. Pour into a bowl or large container. Cover and refrigerate for at least 2 hours.

To serve, pour soup into chilled bowls, and garnish with reserved lime peel.

PYRAMID EQUIVALENT: 2 ½ FRUITS

Nutritional Analysis per Portion

calories 110 ▲ carbohydrate 28 grams ▲ protein 2 grams ▲ fat 0 grams
sodium 13 milligrams ▲ cholesterol 0 milligrams

▲▲

THICKENING TIPS:
LOSE THE FAT, NOT THE BODY

Egg yolks, butter, and cream give soups and sauces their rich, creamy texture. Leaving out those ingredients doesn't mean you are doomed to thin, watery results. Happily you can keep the texture and the flavor without the fat. Here's how:

- ▲ Purée all or part of the soup in a blender or food processor and reheat.
- ▲ Add some leftover mashed potato or dehydrated potato flakes about 10 minutes before the soup is done.
- ▲ Cut a raw potato (sweet or white) into small dice and add at the beginning; it will cook down and add thickness without blending.
- ▲ Stir in a few tablespoons of oatmeal (yes, oatmeal) at the start of cooking.
- ▲ Use evaporated skimmed milk, buttermilk, or nonfat yogurt, with a teaspoon of cornstarch stirred in (one teaspoon for each cup), at the last stage of cooking. Always add cornstarch to cool or room temperature liquids.
- ▲ Mash all or part of the beans used in your recipe.
- ▲ Add raw rice at the start of cooking, or purée some cooked rice and add just before finishing.
- ▲ Toss in bread cubes of any kind about midway through cooking. Varieties such as rye, whole-wheat, or pumpernickel bread will also add a nice hint of flavor.

▲▲

▲▲▲

HANDS-OFF
WHOLE-WHEAT CORNMEAL BREAD

MAKES 1 LOAF; 10 PORTIONS

Since I got a bread machine, there's never a meal or a party at my house without homemade bread. I've always enjoyed making bread from scratch but usually kept it restricted to the cooler winter months. If you don't already own a machine, put one at the top of your wish list—you'll be glad you did.

> 1 1/2 cups EACH bread flour and whole-wheat flour
> 1/2 cup cornmeal
> 1 teaspoon salt
> 1/4 teaspoon ground white pepper
> 1 package active dry yeast*
> 1 cup evaporated skimmed milk
> 1/2 cup water
> 2 tablespoons honey
> 1 tablespoon vegetable oil

Place ingredients in bread pan according to your manufacturer's instructions. Select a LIGHT BREAD setting if the machine has one.

When bread is done, remove it from the pan and place on a wire rack to cool. Store tightly wrapped in aluminum foil.

* Quick-rise yeast works well if your machine has the optional setting.

Conventional Preparation:

If you don't have a bread machine, use "quick-rise" yeast to speed up the rising process; though it requires some manual labor, this bread is worth the effort.

In a medium bowl combine flours. In a large bowl combine half of the flour mixture, cornmeal, salt, pepper, and yeast.

In a small saucepan combine the milk, water, honey, and oil; heat over low heat until liquids are very warm (120° F–130° F). Slowly pour into cornmeal mixture, and, using an electric mixer on medium speed, beat for 2 minutes. Add about half of remaining flour mixture and beat at high speed for 2 minutes, scraping the sides of the bowl occasionally. Stir in remaining flour to make a soft dough. (Add additional bread flour if necessary.)

Turn dough out onto a lightly floured board; knead for 8 to 10 minutes, or until dough is smooth and elastic. Place in a greased bowl, turning to lightly coat top of dough. Cover with a tea towel, and let rise in a warm, draft-free place for about 30 minutes, or until doubled in bulk.

Punch dough down. Let rest; and meanwhile spray a 9 × 5-inch loaf pan with nonstick cooking spray.

Roll dough into a 14 × 9-inch rectangle. Roll up tightly, and tuck edges under loaf. Place in pan, seam-side down. Cover and let rise for about 30 minutes, or until doubled in bulk.

Meanwhile, preheat oven to 375° F. Bake bread for about 35 minutes, or until bread sounds hollow when tapped gently on top. Remove from pan and cool on a wire rack.

PYRAMID EQUIVALENT: 2 BREADS

Nutritional Analysis per Portion

calories 208 ▲ carbohydrate 40 grams ▲ protein 8 grams ▲ fat 2 grams
sodium 252 milligrams ▲ cholesterol 1 milligram

YOGURT-CHIVE BATTER BREAD
WITH POPPY SEEDS

MAKES 1 LOAF; 8 PORTIONS

In less than 2 hours you can make a fragrant yeast bread that doesn't require any kneading. This bread is the ideal introduction to bread baking and lots of fun to make with kids. King Arthur's brand hard white whole-wheat flour (see page 227) works nicely here as a straight substitution. But for other whole-wheat flours, don't use more than a 50-50 blend. After several tests I also opt to use the egg—it makes a far superior loaf and with a yield of eight portions, there's not too much fat or cholesterol per slice.

3¼ cups all-purpose or bread flour
2 packages quick-rise dry yeast
2 teaspoons EACH dried chives and poppy seeds
1 teaspoon salt
1 cup nonfat plain yogurt
½ cup skim milk or water
1 tablespoon EACH vegetable oil and honey
1 egg

In a large mixing bowl combine 1½ cups of the flour, yeast, chives, poppy seeds, and salt; set aside. Spray a 1½ quart casserole with nonstick cooking spray.

In a small saucepan combine the yogurt, milk, oil, and honey, and heat over medium heat for about 3 minutes, until warmed through. (Alternately, place ingredients in a small microwavable dish and heat on MEDIUM-HIGH for 2 minutes.) Pour into flour mixture; add egg.

Using an electric mixer on low speed, beat until just moistened. Increase mixer speed to medium, and beat for 3 minutes, scraping the bowl occasionally. By hand gradually stir in enough of the remaining ¾ cup of flour to make a stiff batter;

scrape batter into prepared casserole. Cover with a kitchen towel, and let rise in a warm place for about 30 minutes, or until doubled.

Meanwhile, preheat oven to 375° F.

Bake for 35 to 40 minutes, or until golden brown. Turn bread onto a wire rack to cool.

Food Processor Preparation:

Insert the metal or dough blade in processor and add all of the flour, yeast, chives, poppy seeds, and salt; pulse to combine. Heat remaining ingredients as directed above. With processor motor running, gradually pour in liquids and egg; mix for 60 seconds. (Note: The batter prepared by this method is quite thick and does not form a ball as conventional dough will.) Scrape batter into prepared casserole, and smooth the top lightly to make an even layer. Proceed as above.

PYRAMID EQUIVALENT: 2 BREADS

Nutritional Analysis per Portion

calories 247 ▲ carbohydrate 45 grams ▲ protein 9 grams ▲ fat 3 grams
sodium 315 milligrams ▲ cholesterol 27 milligrams

▲▲▲

SAVORY PEPPERED CORN MUFFINS

MAKES 12 MUFFINS; 12 PORTIONS

Give your carbohydrate quota a boost with these satisfying and low-fat muffins. Cornmeal, corn, and cooked dried peas toss in a good measure of fiber too. These savory gems are a nice addition to brunch or dinner, not to mention a most satisfying snack. Reduce the salt if sodium is a concern.

1 cup all-purpose flour

1 cup yellow cornmeal

2½ teaspoons baking powder

1¼ teaspoons baking soda

1 teaspoon dried marjoram leaves, crushed

½ teaspoon salt

¼ teaspoon crushed red pepper flakes

1⅓ cups nonfat plain yogurt

1 cup canned cream-style corn

2 tablespoons EACH vegetable oil and honey

1 cup cooked green or yellow dried peas

Preheat oven to 425° F. Spray a 12-cup muffin pan with nonstick cooking spray; set aside.

In a large mixing bowl whisk together the flour, cornmeal, baking powder, baking soda, marjoram, salt, and red pepper.

In a medium bowl whisk together the remaining ingredients, except the peas.

Add the milk mixture and the peas to the flour mixture, and stir until just combined. Do not overmix. Spoon batter into prepared muffin cups.

Bake for 20 to 25 minutes, or until a tester inserted in center of muffins comes out clean. Cool in pan, on a wire rack for 5 minutes. Turn muffins onto rack to finish cooling, or serve warm.

PYRAMID EQUIVALENT: 1 BREAD, ⅓ VEGETABLE

Nutritional Analysis per Portion

calories 162 ▲ carbohydrate 29 grams ▲ protein 5 grams ▲ fat 3 grams

sodium 405 milligrams ▲ cholesterol 1 milligram

▲▲▲

FOCACCIA WITH ONIONS, ROSEMARY, AND FETA CHEESE

MAKES 8 PORTIONS

A classic Italian flat bread, focaccia can be varied at the whim of any cook. This tasty, low-fat version gets its spunk from the distinctive flavor of feta cheese. I like to use a feta with black pepper that's made in Wisconsin. No one can resist the appeal of a warm, freshly baked focaccia—even if you opt to prepare it with a frozen bread loaf. If you're really in a hurry you can skip the onions and merely sprinkle the dough with the cheese and rosemary.

1 tablespoon olive oil, divided
1 cup thinly sliced onion (1 small)
Dough for 1 recipe Pizza Bites (page 74)*
3¹/₂ ounces feta cheese, crumbled (about ¹/₂ cup)
1 ¹/₄ teaspoons dried rosemary, crushed

In a medium skillet heat 2 teaspoons of the oil over medium heat. Add the onions and cook, stirring occasionally until soft; set aside.

Lightly spray an 11 × 7-inch baking pan with nonstick cooking spray. Pat or roll the dough to fit pan; brush with the remaining teaspoon of oil. Spread onions evenly over the dough; sprinkle with the cheese and rosemary.

Cover lightly with a kitchen towel, and let rise in a warm place for about 30 minutes, or until doubled in bulk (or according to package directions). Meanwhile, preheat oven to 350° F.

Bake for 30 minutes, or until puffy and lightly browned. Cut into wedges and serve warm.

* Any brand of unbaked bread dough also works well in this recipe but nonfrozen, refrigerated bread doughs (packaged in a can) generally have more fat than the frozen ones.

PYRAMID EQUIVALENT: 2 BREADS, $\frac{1}{3}$ VEGETABLE, $\frac{1}{4}$ MILK

Nutritional Analysis per Portion

calories 261 ▲ carbohydrate 39 grams ▲ protein 8 grams ▲ fat 8 grams

sodium 334 milligrams ▲ cholesterol 10 milligrams

▲▲

STEAMED CHINESE BUNS

MAKES 8 BUNS; 8 PORTIONS

The minute I saw my dinner guest rip open one of these buns and stuff the Grilled Bangkok Beef Salad (page 149) into it, I knew I had to include the recipe. They are quite easy to make, and quick-rise yeast cuts the time to a fraction. Using a set of stacked bamboo steamers is the authentic way to cook them, but I use the steamer tray in my wok. You could also use a vegetable steamer placed in a large skillet. These buns reheat very well with a few minutes in the steamer.

2$\frac{1}{2}$ cups all-purpose flour
$\frac{1}{2}$ cup hard white whole-wheat flour*
1 package quick-rise yeast
$\frac{1}{2}$ teaspoon salt
1$\frac{1}{4}$ cups very warm water (about 130° F)

In the workbowl of a food processor pulse all ingredients together until just combined. Process for about 1 minute, or until the dough is sticky. Let rest in the workbowl for 10 minutes.

Turn the dough onto a lightly floured board, and roll into a 10-inch log. Cut into 8 pieces. Spray a large platter with nonstick cooking spray, and place the buns about 2 inches apart (use two plates if necessary). Cover with a kitchen towel and let rise for 10 minutes.

* This is King Arthur brand; you can also use regular whole-wheat flour.

Meanwhile bring some water to a boil in a wok or skillet. In two batches, place the buns on steamer trays or rack; cover, and steam for 15 minutes. Turn off heat, and let stand for 1 minute before removing cover.

PYRAMID EQUIVALENT: 2 BREADS

Nutritional Analysis per Portion

calories 170 ▲ carbohydrate 36 grams ▲ protein 5 grams ▲ fat 0 grams
sodium 138 milligrams ▲ cholesterol 0 milligrams

▲▲▲▲▲▲▲▲▲▲▲▲▲▲▲▲▲▲▲▲▲▲▲▲▲▲▲▲▲▲▲▲▲▲▲▲▲▲

SAVORY SIDE DISHES

AROMATIC ASIAN RICE

WEHANI AND BROWN RICE WITH FIGS AND SCALLIONS

MINTY JALAPEÑO RICE SALAD

SHOCKING PINK RICE SALAD

WARM BARLEY-VEGETABLE SALAD

BULGUR WITH LEEKS AND CURRANTS

BULGUR AND BREAD STUFFING

SPICY SCARLET RUNNERS

QUICK 'N' SPICY BLACK-EYED PEAS

LOW-FAT BAKED BEANS

TOMATO BREAD PUDDING

JUICY BAKED BEETS

MUSTARD-LIME BROCCOLI

THAI-STYLE BROCCOLI SLAW

ORANGE-GINGER CARROTS PROVENÇAL

SPINACH WITH GARLIC AND RAISINS

SHREDDED SPROUTS WITH RED PEPPER AND DILL

TROPICAL SUCCOTASH SAUTÉ

CREAMY MASHED POTATOES

LIVELY TWO-TONE POTATO SALAD

VEGETABLE TORTILLA ROLLS

▲▲▲

With its emphasis on grains, breads, fruits and vegetables, the Food Guide Pyramid gives new meaning to side dishes. Unless the main part of the meal is a hearty soup, a lasagna, or chili, side dishes are needed to fill in for the copious amounts of meat and fats many people are used to eating. In fact, this section can provide you with an opportunity to create a meatless meal by serving three or four side dishes at the same time.

The recipes here make it easy. There is an ample collection from which to choose. Creamy Mashed Potatoes may seem familiar to you. In making them, however, you'll immediately notice the cutback in butter and milk, but I promise you'll never miss it in the tasting. Some people may not have tried bulgur yet. This nutty-tasting whole grain is the underpinning of Bulgur with Leeks and Currants, a sumptuous and satisfying dish. Another recipe, Bulgur and Bread Stuffing, is strengthened with the addition of bulgur when the fat—which is plentiful in many traditional stuffings—is whittled down to a minimum. With its grated beet, Shocking Pink Rice Salad will be the center of attention whenever you serve it. And the blend of flavors in it belie the total absence of fat. Tomato Bread Pudding is comfort food at its best. Soft, warm, and moist, it is gently seasoned with onion and basil. It can be prepared with either fresh or canned tomatoes, and either way you get a nice boost of vitamin C.

You won't be at a loss for ways to put more vegetables on your table either. Mustard-Lime Broccoli is fragrant with the Indian influence of cumin, cinnamon, and coriander. Then you'll have lots of fun recycling the broccoli stalks from that recipe to make Thai-Style Broccoli Slaw, another delicious fat-free dish. If you haven't tried chayote—a trendy, tropical summer squash—Tropical Succotash Sauté is an ideal introduction. You'll be amazed at how delectable this medley is despite the fact that only two teaspoons of butter are used to make it.

Getting your 5 a Day allotment won't be hard with other recipes like Spinach with Garlic and Raisins. Fashioned after a Catalan dish, it's loaded with beta carotene but relieved of the fat that's traditionally used. Juicy Baked Beets, wrapped in foil with a splash of orange juice, puts these jewels back on the menu with no effort at all.

This chapter is a good way to choose more generously from the base of the Pyramid—breads and grains—and step right up to the next level of fruits and vegetables. Both of these categories are good sources of fiber, as well as important nutrients like vitamin C and beta carotene. What you won't find here is lots of added fat.

▲▲▲

AROMATIC ASIAN RICE

MAKES 4 PORTIONS

For those who like a delicate side dish, this fragrant rice couldn't be easier to prepare. Cinnamon sticks and cloves give it soft undertones and the kind of versatility that make it a nice complement to many meals. Jasmine rice, now in many supermarkets and in Asian markets, or any other aromatic rice such as Basmati or Texmati, lends a distinctive touch.

    2 cups water
    1 cup uncooked rice, preferably jasmine
    1 teaspoon vegetable oil or butter
    1/4 teaspoon salt
    1 1/2 cinnamon sticks, about 3 inches long
    4 whole cloves

In a medium saucepan combine all the ingredients; bring to a boil. Reduce heat, cover, and simmer for about 20 minutes, or until the water is absorbed. Remove cinnamon sticks and cloves. Fluff with a fork and serve.

Microwave Preparation:

In a 2-quart microwavable casserole combine all the ingredients. Microwave, uncovered, on HIGH for 10 to 12 minutes, until about two-thirds of the water is absorbed, and there are steamy bubbles on top; stir twice.

Cover with a lid or vented plastic wrap. Microwave on HIGH for 10 to 12 minutes, or until most of the water is absorbed. Let stand, covered, for 5 minutes. Fluff with a fork and serve.

PYRAMID EQUIVALENT: 1½ BREADS

Nutritional Analysis per Portion

calories 180 ▲ carbohydrate 37 grams ▲ protein 3 grams ▲ fat 1 gram
sodium 138 milligrams ▲ cholesterol 0 milligrams

▲▲▲

WEHANI AND BROWN RICE WITH FIGS AND SCALLIONS

MAKES 4 PORTIONS

Wehani is a naturally aromatic brown rice. I like it because it's a unique and attractive rust-colored long-grain brown rice that fills your kitchen with the aroma of buttered popcorn. It's fun to mix Wehani rice with brown rice, and/or barley, which both take about the same amount of time to cook. For this recipe, I especially like to use dried Calimyrna figs from California, but Mission or any of your favorites are fine, too. Slice some of the green tops of the scallions very thin, and sprinkle them over the top of this dish just before serving to make it more colorful.

2 teaspoons vegetable oil
1/2 cup thinly sliced scallions (green onions)
3/4 cup EACH Wehani and brown rice
1 1/2 cups EACH water and orange juice
1/2 cup chopped dried figs
1/8 teaspoon ground red pepper

In a 3-quart saucepan heat oil over medium heat. Add scallions and cook, stirring occasionally, for 2 minutes; stir in rices and cook 1 minute longer. Add water, orange juice, and figs, and bring to a boil. Cover, reduce heat, and simmer for about 40 minutes, or until most of the liquid is absorbed and the rices are tender. Add pepper; fluff with a fork and serve.

PYRAMID EQUIVALENT: 2 1/4 BREADS, 1 FRUIT, 1/4 VEGETABLE

Nutritional Analysis per Portion

calories 386 ▲ carbohydrate 80 grams ▲ protein 7 grams ▲ fat 5 grams
sodium 11 milligrams ▲ cholesterol 0 milligrams

▲▲

MINTY JALAPEÑO RICE SALAD

MAKES 4 PORTIONS

Sweet peas smooth the fire of the jalapeño pepper in this zesty rice salad. Brown rice gives it a nice nutty flavor. With everything this salad has going for it, you'll never miss the fat. Remove the seeds from the jalapeño if you want a milder-flavored salad.

5 cups cooked brown rice

1 10-ounce package petit peas, defrosted and drained (about 2 cups)

3 scallions (green onions), including green tops, sliced thin

1 small jalapeño pepper, sliced thin

1/2 cup EACH loosely packed parsley and cilantro leaves, chopped fine

1/3 cup loosely packed mint leaves, chopped fine

Juice of 2 large lemons

1 1/2 tablespoons Dijon mustard

Salt and freshly ground black pepper to taste

In a large bowl combine the rice, peas, scallions, pepper, parsley, cilantro, and mint.

In a small bowl combine the lemon juice and mustard. Pour the dressing over the rice mixture and stir until thoroughly combined. Add salt and pepper to taste.

PYRAMID EQUIVALENT: 2 1/2 BREADS, 1 1/4 VEGETABLES

Nutritional Analysis per Portion

calories 339 ▲ carbohydrate 69 grams ▲ protein 10 grams ▲ fat 3 grams
sodium 282 milligrams ▲ cholesterol 0 milligrams

▲▲

SHOCKING PINK RICE SALAD

MAKES 4 PORTIONS

Grated beet gives a brilliant red tone to this brown rice salad. It's an eye-catching dish that contains no fat at all. If you're making it the night before, do not add the vinegar, lemon juice, salt, and red pepper until the next day; stir them in about an hour before serving.

4 cups cooked brown rice

¼ cup thinly sliced scallions (green onions), white part and about 1 inch of
   the green tops

6 large basil leaves, sliced thin

½ cup finely grated raw beet (not necessary to peel)

¾ cup diced zucchini

3 tablespoons rice vinegar

2 tablespoons lemon juice

¼ teaspoon salt

¼ teaspoon ground red pepper

Combine all the ingredients in a large bowl. Adjust seasonings to taste. Cover and refrigerate.

Let stand at room temperature for about an hour before serving.

PYRAMID EQUIVALENT: 2 BREADS, ¾ VEGETABLE

Nutritional Analysis per Portion

calories 234 ▲ carbohydrate 49 grams ▲ protein 6 grams ▲ fat 2 grams
sodium 162 milligrams ▲ cholesterol 0 milligrams

▲▲

WARM BARLEY-VEGETABLE SALAD

MAKES 6 PORTIONS

The wonderful blend of flavors, textures, and colors belies the virtual absence of oil in this salad. It is quite simple to prepare and an excellent reason for keeping a batch of cooked barley in the freezer. Serve it warm or chilled.

$^1/_2$ cup chopped onion

$^1/_4$ cup vegetable broth or water (see page 40)

$^3/_4$ teaspoon dried thyme, crumbled

$^1/_4$ teaspoon crushed red pepper flakes, or to taste

4 cups coarsely chopped zucchini, patty pan, or summer squash (about
    1 $^1/_4$ pounds)

3 cups cooked barley

1 $^1/_2$ cups chopped tomatoes

$^1/_4$ cup chopped fresh cilantro

2 tablespoons fresh lime juice

$^1/_4$ teaspoon salt

In a large skillet or wok combine the onion, 2 tablespoons of the broth or water, thyme, and pepper flakes, and cook over medium-high heat for 10 minutes, or until onion is tender and just begins to brown, stirring occasionally. Add the remaining broth or water, the squash, and barley; cover and cook for about 5 minutes or until squash is tender-crisp. Add remaining ingredients and stir thoroughly to combine. Serve, or re-cover and refrigerate. Bring almost to room temperature before serving.

PYRAMID EQUIVALENT: 1 BREAD, 2 VEGETABLES

Nutritional Analysis per Portion

calories 128 ▲ carbohydrate 29 grams ▲ protein 3 grams ▲ fat 0 grams
sodium 100 milligrams ▲ cholesterol 0 milligrams

▲▲

BULGUR WITH LEEKS AND CURRANTS

MAKES 4 PORTIONS

Bulgur is a nutty-tasting grain with a tender, chewy texture. Often used in Middle Eastern dishes, it's at home as a salad, as a side dish, or in casseroles for a main dish, and it is often added to soups. This tasty side dish calls for a medium grind of bulgur.

> 2 teaspoons vegetable oil
> 1 cup thoroughly washed and thinly sliced leeks (white and about 1 inch of the green top)
> 1 1/2 cups medium bulgur
> 1/4 cup currants
> 3 cups chicken broth (see page 40)
> 1/2 teaspoon salt
> 1/8 teaspoon EACH ground nutmeg and ground white pepper

In a 3-quart saucepan heat oil over medium heat. Add leeks and cook, stirring occasionally, for 2 minutes; stir in remaining ingredients and bring to a boil.

Cover, reduce heat, and simmer for 15 to 20 minutes, or until most of the liquid is absorbed. Fluff with a fork and adjust seasonings if necessary.

PYRAMID EQUIVALENT: 3 3/4 BREADS, 1/4 VEGETABLE, 1/4 FRUIT

Nutritional Analysis per Portion

calories 264 ▴ carbohydrate 51 grams ▴ protein 9 grams ▴ fat 4 grams
sodium 328 milligrams ▴ cholesterol 0 milligrams

▴▴

BULGUR AND BREAD STUFFING

MAKES 10 PORTIONS

Traditional stuffings essentially start out from a wholesome combination of ingredients including breads and grains with vegetables like onions, celery, and carrots. The addition of butter, cream, eggs, sausage, bacon, and nuts then turns them into a fat and cholesterol overload. This delicately sweetened yet very savory stuffing is a low-fat, cholesterol-free blend of bulgur and sourdough bread (or any favorite bread of yours), combined with dried apricots, orange juice, herbs, and a touch of ground red pepper (cayenne).

Here is an ideal dish in which to use frozen egg substitutes. The egg is only being used as a binder and the substitutes have no fat or cholesterol. The recipe can easily be cut in half or doubled: remember that tightly wrapped stuffing freezes well. The stuffing can be served as a side dish for vegetarians if you make it with vegetable stock instead of the chicken broth. Use it to stuff vegetables like sweet bell peppers and winter squashes for a meatless entrée or as a traditional stuffing baked outside the bird.

1 1/3 cups coarse or medium bulgur
2 cups boiling water
2 tablespoons olive oil
2 cups coarsely chopped onion
2 cups sliced celery
6 cups stale sourdough bread, cut into cubes (about 8 ounces)
2 cups chicken or vegetable broth (see page 40)
1 cup orange juice
1 cup frozen egg substitute (equivalent to 4 whole eggs), thawed
1 1/2 cups chopped dried apricots (about 8 ounces)
1/2 cup chopped fresh Italian (flat-leaf) parsley
1 tablespoon chopped fresh thyme, or 1 1/2 teaspoons dried thyme leaves, crumbled
2 teaspoons chopped fresh sage or 1 teaspoon dried rubbed sage (not ground sage)
1/4 teaspoon ground red pepper

Preheat oven to 350° F. Spray a 13 × 9-inch baking pan with nonstick cooking spray; set aside.

Place the bulgur in a large mixing bowl; pour boiling water over it. Cover tightly with plastic wrap and set aside for about 20 minutes.

In a large nonstick skillet heat the oil over medium-high heat. Add the onions and celery and cook, stirring occasionally, for about 8 minutes, or until the onion is translucent. Cool slightly.

Fluff the bulgur with a fork; add the cooked vegetables and the remaining ingredients. Stir thoroughly until blended; add additional broth and juice if mixture appears dry. Transfer dressing to prepared pan; smooth to make an even layer. Cover with aluminum foil, and bake for 20 minutes; remove foil and bake for another 15 minutes, until dressing is browned on top.

PYRAMID EQUIVALENT: 1 1/3 BREADS, 3/4 VEGETABLE, 3/4 FRUIT

Nutritional Analysis per Portion

calories 249 ▴ carbohydrate 47 grams ▴ protein 8 grams ▴ fat 4 grams
sodium 209 milligrams ▴ cholesterol 0 milligrams

▴▴

SPICY SCARLET RUNNERS

MAKES 4 PORTIONS

Scarlet runner beans are among the wide variety of domestic dried beans that have appeared on the market over the last few years. These deep red beans have small black markings and are a bit larger and flatter than kidney beans. The seasonings here go well with just about any bean of your choice. If you're using canned beans, Eden brand has an excellent line of canned organic beans that are packed with no added salt.

3 cups cooked scarlet runner beans (or other large beans), or 3 cups
    canned beans, rinsed and drained
1 medium jalapeño pepper (including seeds), chopped fine
2 garlic cloves, minced
2 tablespoons balsamic vinegar
1 tablespoon EACH olive oil and fresh lime juice
2 teaspoons Dijon mustard
1/4 teaspoon salt

In a medium bowl combine all ingredients until blended. Cover, and chill until ready to serve. Adjust seasonings to taste, if necessary.

PYRAMID EQUIVALENT: 1½ VEGETABLES

Nutritional Analysis per Portion

calories 225 ▲ carbohydrate 35 grams ▲ protein 13 grams ▲ fat 4 grams
sodium 219 milligrams ▲ cholesterol 0 milligrams

▲▲

QUICK 'N' SPICY BLACK-EYED PEAS

MAKES 6 PORTIONS

Black-eyed peas are traditionally eaten on New Year's Day in the South as a symbol of health and prosperity to come. Unlike other legumes, black-eyed peas don't need to be presoaked if you're inclined to make them from scratch. You might also want to look in the produce section for a precooked variety from Frieda's that takes just about 15 minutes to cook. Remove the seeds from the jalapeño pepper for a milder dish.

1½ teaspoons extra-virgin olive oil
1 cup sliced mushrooms
½ cup finely chopped onions
½ cup finely chopped celery (including leaves)
1 medium jalapeño pepper, chopped fine
4 cups cooked black-eyed peas or canned beans, rinsed and drained
¾ teaspoon dried thyme, crumbled
⅛ teaspoon crushed red pepper flakes, optional
Pinch nutmeg
2 to 3 tablespoons balsamic vinegar

In a large saucepan, heat oil over medium-high heat. Stir in the mushrooms, onions, celery, and jalapeño pepper. Cook for 5 minutes, stirring occasionally; add the remaining ingredients. Cover and cook over medium heat for 5 minutes.

PYRAMID EQUIVALENT: 1½ VEGETABLES

Nutritional Analysis per Portion

calories 104 ▲ carbohydrate 17 grams ▲ protein 6 grams ▲ fat 2 grams
sodium 195 milligrams ▲ cholesterol 0 milligrams

▲▲

LOW-FAT BAKED BEANS

MAKES 6 PORTIONS
(ABOUT 1½ QUARTS)

With just about one-half teaspoon of oil per serving, these beans offer practically guilt-free enjoyment. They are also made without any meat at all. The recipe—sent to me by Pat Mason, a food writer friend in Maine—calls for beans to be made in a slow cooker, or Crock-Pot. Based on the reactions I got, the final result is worth the price of the cooker. (Besides, if you look in the back of the cupboard, chances are that many of you already own this convenient appliance!)

Liquid smoke makes up for the flavor lost when the traditional salt pork is omitted, and it also fills the kitchen with a wonderful aroma. Unlike other conventional recipes, the beans don't need any presoaking or precooking here.

5 cups water
2½ cups (1 pound) dry beans (pinto, kidney, black, etc., or any combination), rinsed and drained
1 tablespoon canola or other vegetable oil
1 tablespoon natural hickory seasoning (liquid smoke)
1½ cups coarsely chopped onion
¼ cup packed brown sugar
1½ teaspoons salt

In a slow cooker combine 4 cups of the water and the remaining ingredients, except the salt. Cover and cook on HIGH for 4 hours, or until the beans are tender, adding the remaining cup of water halfway through cooking. When the beans are cooked, add the salt.

PYRAMID EQUIVALENT: 2 VEGETABLES
(OR ½ VEGETABLE AND 1¾ OUNCES MEAT ALTERNATE)

Nutritional Analysis per Portion

calories 327 ▲ carbohydrate 60 grams ▲ protein 16 grams ▲ fat 3 grams
sodium 560 milligrams ▲ cholesterol 0 milligrams

▲▲

TOMATO BREAD PUDDING

MAKES 6 PORTIONS

This soft, savory pudding was inspired by a recipe Frank Arcuri, a talented natural foods chef, included in an article he wrote for *Food Arts* magazine.

9 ounces sourdough or other crusty bread (about 7 cups), cut or torn into
    2-inch pieces
1½ tablespoons extra-virgin olive oil
1½ cups chopped onion
2 tablespoons EACH chopped fresh basil and Italian (flat-leaf) parsley
1 tablespoon chopped oil-cured olives (about 8 small)
⅛ teaspoon crushed red pepper flakes, or to taste
3 cups canned no-salt-added crushed tomatoes*
⅓ cup grated Parmesan cheese (see page 41), optional

* You may substitute 3 cups chopped plum tomatoes (about 2 pounds) for the canned tomatoes.

Preheat oven to 350° F. Spray an 11 × 7-inch baking dish with nonstick cooking spray; set aside.

Moisten the bread cubes briefly in water; squeeze dry and set aside.

In a large nonstick skillet heat oil over medium heat, add remaining ingredients, except tomatoes and cheese, and cook for about 5 minutes, or until the onions are tender. Remove from heat; add the bread and tomatoes; stir well to combine. Spoon mixture into baking dish; sprinkle with cheese, if desired.

Cover with aluminum foil, and bake for 20 minutes; remove foil and bake for 5 minutes longer, or until golden brown. Cut into wedges and serve.

PYRAMID EQUIVALENT: 1½ BREADS, 1½ VEGETABLES

Nutritional Analysis per Portion

calories 193 ▲ carbohydrate 31 grams ▲ protein 5 grams ▲ fat 6 grams
sodium 325 milligrams ▲ cholesterol 0 milligrams

▲▲

JUICY BAKED BEETS

MAKES 4 PORTIONS

I'm a great fan of beets. They're so versatile, low in calories, and extraordinarily delicious when they're fresh. I can't understand why more people aren't eating them frequently. With only 55 calories per cup, moderate amounts of vitamins A and C, and some potassium, they should be high on your list too.

Use larger beets here if you can find them—figure one per person. Though I prefer them just sprinkled with a bit of salt and pepper, you can also toss in a pinch of dried thyme, marjoram, or dill just before wrapping, or perk them up with a few tablespoons of fresh orange juice as below.

4 large beets, scrubbed and trimmed (about 2 pounds)
½ cup orange juice
Salt and ground white pepper, optional

Preheat oven to 375° F.

Wrap each beet tightly in aluminum foil, sprinkling each one with about 2 tablespoons orange juice before closing the foil. Place directly on oven rack, and bake for 1 to 1¼ hours, or until tender when pierced to the center with the tip of a sharp knife.

Carefully open each packet and sprinkle with salt and pepper, if desired.

Serve beets with their juices, in aluminum foil if desired.

PYRAMID EQUIVALENT: 2 VEGETABLES

Nutritional Analysis per Portion

calories 81 ▲ carbohydrate 19 grams ▲ protein 2 grams ▲ fat 0 grams
sodium 110 milligrams ▲ cholesterol 0 milligrams

▲▲

MUSTARD-LIME BROCCOLI

MAKES 6 PORTIONS

Food writer Julie Sahni inspired this fragrant broccoli dish. She believes that microwave cooking is the best way to cook broccoli, and so it is done here. (Her book *Mogul Microwave* is an outstanding work that makes Indian cooking simple and fast.) I also believe that microwaving intensifies flavors while retaining great color and crispness in vegetables.

This recipe provides a good opportunity to recycle broccoli stems and try the Thai-Style Broccoli Slaw (page 107).

2 pounds broccoli

$^1/_2$ cup thinly sliced onion

$^3/_4$ cup chicken broth *or* vegetable broth (see page 40)

2 teaspoons peanut or vegetable oil

1$^1/_4$ teaspoons dry mustard

1 teaspoon EACH ground cumin, cuminseed, and ground coriander

$^1/_8$ teaspoon EACH ground cinnamon and ground red pepper

2 tablespoons fresh lime juice

Trim broccoli. Cut off stalks and reserve for another use. Cut florets into bite-size pieces (you should have about 7 cups); set aside.

In a large microwavable skillet or casserole combine the remaining ingredients, except the lime juice.

Microwave on HIGH, uncovered, for 2 minutes. Add the reserved florets in batches, stirring thoroughly to coat with spice mixture. Cover with a lid or vented plastic wrap. Microwave on HIGH for 5 to 7 minutes, or until broccoli is tender-crisp, stirring once during cooking. Let stand for 2 minutes. Sprinkle lime juice over the top and serve.

Stovetop Preparation:

Follow directions above using a large skillet. Cook onion and spices for 5 minutes. Add the remaining ingredients, except lime juice, cover and cook for 10 to 12 minutes, or until the broccoli is tender. Add lime juice and serve.

PYRAMID EQUIVALENT: 2 VEGETABLES

Nutritional Analysis per Portion

calories 54 ▲ carbohydrate 7 grams ▲ protein 3 grams ▲ fat 2 grams
sodium 33 milligrams ▲ cholesterol 0 milligrams

▲▲

THAI-STYLE BROCCOLI SLAW

MAKES 4 PORTIONS

What do you do with all those broccoli stems when a recipe calls for broccoli florets? Maybe you use them for vegetable stock, or slice them diagonally and serve them raw for hors d'oeuvres, or you probably just toss them out like most people do. Here is a good alternative.

Put your food processor to work, or pull out a grater and try this spicy Asian side dish. You can also scout the produce section for preshredded packages of broccoli stalks. Rice vinegar adds a slight sweetness to the slaw that is common in many Thai dishes.

    4 large broccoli stems (from about 2 pounds broccoli), trimmed and lightly
        peeled
    1 large carrot, peeled
    ¼ cup rice vinegar
    2 teaspoons fish sauce (nam pla)*
    1 teaspoon minced garlic
    ⅛ teaspoon crushed red pepper flakes, or to taste

Use the fine shredding blade in your food processor or a hand grater to shred the broccoli and carrot (you should have about 4 cups of broccoli and 1 cup of carrot).

In a large bowl toss all ingredients together until combined. Cover and refrigerate for 2 to 4 hours to let flavors blend.

* Available in Asian markets or in the ethnic foods section in some supermarkets.

PYRAMID EQUIVALENT: 2 ½ VEGETABLES

Nutritional Analysis per Portion

calories 52 ▲ carbohydrate 10 grams ▲ protein 4 grams ▲ fat 1 gram
sodium 42 milligrams ▲ cholesterol 0 milligrams

▲▲▲

ORANGE-GINGER CARROTS PROVENÇAL

MAKES 4 PORTIONS

Orange juice, fresh ginger, and carrots are one of those felicitous combinations I'm reluctant to disturb. But adding some oil-cured olives gives an interesting touch to this high-fiber vegetable, also rich in vitamin A and beta carotene. I also make this with chicken or vegetable broth instead of the water, if I have it on hand.

 1/4 cup EACH orange juice and water
 2 teaspoons sweet butter
 1 1/2 teaspoons chopped fresh ginger
 1 pound carrots, scraped and cut into 1/2-inch slices
 2 tablespoons pitted and chopped oil-cured Italian olives
 1/4 teaspoon freshly ground black pepper

In a medium saucepan or skillet combine the orange juice, water, butter, and ginger; bring to a boil. Add the carrots. Reduce heat to medium-low; cover, and cook for 10 minutes, or until the carrots are tender. Stir in the olives and pepper.

PYRAMID EQUIVALENT: 1 1/4 VEGETABLES

Nutritional Analysis per Portion

calories 83 ▲ carbohydrate 12 grams ▲ protein 1 gram ▲ fat 4 grams
sodium 183 milligrams ▲ cholesterol 5 milligrams

▲▲

SPINACH WITH GARLIC AND RAISINS

MAKES 4 PORTIONS

Based on a classic Catalan dish, this recipe uses vinegar to lift the flavors. It's very easy to make and a most pleasant way to boost your vegetable intake.

$1/3$ cup chicken stock or water (see page 40)
2 tablespoons balsamic vinegar
2 teaspoons olive oil
$1/3$ cup raisins or currants
4 garlic cloves, minced
$1/4$ teaspoon ground nutmeg
$1 1/2$ pounds fresh spinach, trimmed and washed (about 10 cups)

In a large nonstick skillet or wok combine all the ingredients except the spinach; bring to a boil. Add the spinach and toss together for about 2 minutes, or until the spinach is just wilted.

PYRAMID EQUIVALENT: $2 1/2$ VEGETABLES, $1/4$ FRUIT

Nutritional Analysis per Portion

calories 92 ▲ carbohydrate 15 grams ▲ protein 4 grams ▲ fat 3 grams
sodium 103 milligrams ▲ cholesterol 0 milligrams

▲▲

SHREDDED SPROUTS WITH RED PEPPER AND DILL

MAKES 4 PORTIONS

Brussels sprouts are not high on the list of favorite vegetables for most people. But I discovered that serving them sliced thin gets rave reviews every time. I am giving this recipe for cooking in the microwave; not only is the technique easy, but it also seems to eliminate the cabbagey flavor that people dislike. It helps to know that these little plants are a source of vitamin C and also contain some vitamin A, beta carotene, thiamine, iron, potassium, and phosphorus.

1 pound Brussels sprouts, trimmed and tough outer leaves removed; thinly
     sliced crosswise
$\frac{1}{2}$ cup chopped red bell pepper
$\frac{1}{4}$ cup chopped fresh dill
$\frac{1}{3}$ cup chicken stock or water (see page 40)
1 tablespoon Dijon mustard
2 teaspoons sweet butter
$\frac{1}{4}$ teaspoon freshly ground black pepper

In a 2-quart microwavable casserole, toss all the ingredients together using a fork until combined and most of the Brussels sprouts are separated. Cover partially with lid or with vented plastic wrap. Microwave on HIGH for 5 to 7 minutes, or until the Brussels sprouts are tender.

Stir and re-cover. Let stand for 2 minutes.

PYRAMID EQUIVALENT: 2 $\frac{1}{2}$ VEGETABLES

Nutritional Analysis per Portion

calories 74 ▲ carbohydrate 11 grams ▲ protein 4 grams ▲ fat 3 grams
sodium 144 milligrams ▲ cholesterol 5 milligrams

TROPICAL SUCCOTASH SAUTÉ

MAKES 4 PORTIONS

Here's a good way to introduce chayote, a tropical summer squash from Latin America, to your menu. Now grown in California, Florida, and Louisiana, this gourdlike fruit is about the size and shape of a large pear, with a white, mild-tasting flesh beneath its pale green skin. It's found in most supermarkets throughout the year, though its peak is in the winter months. If you can't find chayote, you can substitute zucchini.

A smidgen of butter adds a rich flavor to this combination of ingredients that is often called succotash. We don't often think of buying fresh corn on the cob except in the summer months, but Golden Sweet fresh corn is available all year long, and it's superb.

2 teaspoons unsalted butter
1 large chayote, peeled, seeded, and cut into ¹/₂-inch pieces (about
    1¹/₂ cups)
2 ears fresh corn, husked and kernels removed, or 2 cups frozen kernels,
    defrosted
1 cup cooked lima beans or 1 cup frozen baby limas, defrosted
¹/₂ cup chopped red bell pepper
¹/₄ teaspoon EACH salt and freshly ground black pepper

In a large nonstick skillet, melt butter over medium-high heat; add chayote and cook, stirring occasionally, for 2 minutes. Add remaining ingredients, except salt and pepper, and stir well to combine. Cover and reduce heat to medium-low. Cook for about 5 minutes, or until vegetables are tender. Add salt and pepper, and serve.

PYRAMID EQUIVALENT: 2¹/₂ VEGETABLES

Nutritional Analysis per Portion

calories 150 ▲ carbohydrate 28 grams ▲ protein 6 grams ▲ fat 3 grams
sodium 157 milligrams ▲ cholesterol 5 milligrams

▲▲

CREAMY MASHED POTATOES

MAKES 4 PORTIONS

Russet potatoes, with their high starch content, are what most folks use for making mashed potatoes. But I like to use the Yukon Gold when cutting down on butter and milk because they have a waxy, almost creamy texture. Here nonfat cottage cheese with a bit of skim milk and just a tablespoon of butter makes a rich-tasting comfort food. Like some trendy chefs, you might want to use olive oil instead of butter.

1 3/4 pounds Yukon Gold potatoes, peeled and cut into cubes
1/2 cup EACH nonfat cottage cheese and skim milk
1 tablespoon sweet butter or olive oil
1/2 teaspoon salt
Freshly ground black pepper

In a medium saucepan cover the potatoes with cold water. Partially cover, bring to a boil, and cook for about 15 minutes, or until the potatoes are tender.

Meanwhile, in a blender liquefy the cottage cheese and milk.

Drain the potatoes and return them to the pot. Using an electric mixer on medium speed or a potato masher, mash potatoes until almost smooth. Turn heat on low and slowly stir in cottage cheese mixture. Add butter, salt, and pepper to taste.

PYRAMID EQUIVALENT: 1 VEGETABLE

Nutritional Analysis per Portion

calories 204 ▲ carbohydrate 35 grams ▲ protein 8 grams ▲ fat 3 grams
sodium 404 milligrams ▲ cholesterol 11 milligrams

▲▲

LIVELY TWO-TONE POTATO SALAD

MAKES 4 PORTIONS

Yams make a nice addition to potato salad, and they're a good source of beta carotene. You can use any combination of your favorite herbs—dill, chives, or chervil—in place of the ones here. There's barely any fat in this potato salad. It's so guiltless, you can serve it often.

1¼ pounds small red (new) potatoes (about 12)
1 pound yams (2 medium)
3 scallions (green onions), including green tops, sliced thin
½ cup EACH loosely packed parsley and cilantro leaves, chopped fine
⅓ cup loosely packed mint leaves, chopped fine
½ cup EACH nonfat plain yogurt and reduced-calorie mayonnaise
¼ teaspoon Tabasco sauce
Juice of 1 large lemon
Salt and freshly ground black pepper to taste

Preheat oven to 375° F.

Wash and scrub the potatoes and yams. Bake until just tender. Let cool slightly and cut into 1-inch cubes, leaving skins on.

In a large mixing bowl combine the potatoes, yams, scallions, and chopped herbs.

In a small bowl combine the remaining ingredients, except the salt and pepper, until well blended. Stir the sauce into the potato mixture.

Sprinkle with salt and pepper to taste and adjust seasonings if desired.

PYRAMID EQUIVALENT: 2 VEGETABLES

Nutritional Analysis per Portion

calories 338 ▲ carbohydrate 60 grams ▲ protein 7 grams ▲ fat 8 grams
sodium 212 milligrams ▲ cholesterol 10 milligrams

▲▲▲

VEGETABLE TORTILLA ROLLS

MAKES 2 PORTIONS

This vegetable roll is an adaptation of one served at Arizona 206, a southwestern restaurant in New York City. I am especially fond of whole-wheat tortillas, with their slightly sweet, nutty flavor. You can toss the vegetables with any of your favorite dressings—I sometimes even use salsa. Using the fine shredding blade of the food processor gives the vegetable a delicate touch. With some fruit and a wedge of cheese it makes a nice luncheon or light dinner meal.

    3 cups finely grated vegetables (such as red and white cabbage, carrot,
        radicchio, jicama, celery, and broccoli stalks)
    1/3 cup Apricot Vinaigrette (page 125)
    2 10-inch whole-wheat tortillas

In a large bowl toss vegetables and dressing until combined.

   Heat a medium nonstick skillet, and lightly toast each tortilla on both sides over medium heat. Mound half the vegetable mixture across the bottom half of each tortilla, fold in the sides, and roll up. Place two toothpicks about 2 inches apart in the center of each roll; slice diagonally and serve.

PYRAMID EQUIVALENT: 2 BREADS, 3 VEGETABLES

Nutritional Analysis per Portion

calories 272 ▲ carbohydrate 43 grams ▲ protein 7 grams ▲ fat 9 grams
sodium 296 milligrams ▲ cholesterol 0 milligrams

▲▲

SALADS, DRESSINGS, SAUCES, AND BROTHS

CHILLED ASPARAGUS AND GRAPE SALAD

ITALIAN BREAD SALAD

SPINACH, CITRUS, AND GOAT CHEESE SALAD

SESAME-DRESSED FIELD GREENS WITH APPLES AND WATER CHESTNUTS

LEMONY DILL DRESSING

CILANTRO-LIME DRESSING

HONEY-DIJON DRESSING

SESAME DRESSING

APRICOT VINAIGRETTE

CREAMY TARRAGON DRESSING

▲▲▲

When it comes to the idea of "healthy" foods, salads are one of the first that come to mind. Nearly all of the usual ingredients—vegetables, fruits, grains, lean meats, seafood, etc.—imply fresh and wholesome food. For the most part that's what salads are. But when it comes to the dressing, a nutritional disaster may be at hand.

I often watch people in a restaurant scrupulously order salad dressing "on the side." Then, in a flash, every last drop of it is poured over the top, or perhaps spooned on in two or three stages until it's all used up. Sometimes I think they have used more than any waitperson would have ladled on in the first place. The problem is that most salad dressings contain about 90 calories per tablespoon. It's not unreasonable to estimate that these "side" portions may add up to as much as half a cup—or 8 tablespoons—and can equal over 700 calories that consist primarily of fat! Remember the advice at the tip of the Pyramid: use fats and oils "sparingly."

In this chapter I am going to show you lots of ways to prepare salad dressings that are delicious and light in fat and calories. Most of the oil traditionally used is replaced with juice, nectar, or broth. Adding some extra herbs and spices is a good way to fool the palate about the change. I hope these recipes will inspire you to create your own once you discover how good they are.

Use just enough dressing to lightly coat the salad. Allow for two tablespoons of dressing per person. Thoroughly tossing the ingredients in a large bowl helps you to use less dressing. To enhance the flavor, first rub the inside of the empty bowl with a cut clove of garlic.

If you like a thick, rich dressing try the Creamy Tarragon Dressing. It is made with nonfat yogurt and reduced-calorie mayonnaise but tastes like a sour-cream dressing. Apricot nectar gives extra smoothness to the Apricot Vinaigrette so that you never miss the relatively large quantity of oil that's generally included in dressings of this type.

Try your hand at making stock from scratch. It's really quite simple and far superior to any broth you pour from a can. Homemade stock is also an efficient way to use up vegetables that are waning in the refrigerator, and recycle a chicken (or turkey) carcass.

Have a look at the Easy Tomato Sauce when tomatoes are abundant and flavorful. It's very easy to make, and like stock, freezes well. When you're in a hurry, or the tomatoes are bland and flat-tasting, Quick Tomato Sauce is the answer. This one takes only 20 minutes to cook and requires very little effort.

▲▲▲

CHILLED ASPARAGUS AND GRAPE SALAD

MAKES 4 PORTIONS

This simple salad makes a stunning presentation and is also a perfect make-ahead appetizer. It's a nice contribution to filling your 5 a Day quota. Try to find slender, pencil-thin asparagus for this dish.

  1 pound slender asparagus, washed and trimmed
  1/2 cup julienne-cut red bell pepper
  1 cup green and red seedless grapes, halved
  1/2 cup Apricot Vinaigrette (page 125)

Place a vegetable steamer rack in a large skillet or Dutch oven filled with about 1 inch of boiling water. Lay asparagus on top. Cover and cook about 5 minutes, or until just tender. Place pepper strips over the asparagus. Cover 1 minute longer (off the heat).

Carefully remove steamer rack and blanch vegetables under cold running water. Drain, and chill until ready to serve.

Distribute asparagus evenly among four chilled salad plates, fanning them out in a semicircle; scatter a few strips of red pepper on top. Place about ½ cup of grapes at the base of the asparagus. Drizzle 1 to 2 tablespoons of dressing over the top of each plate.

Microwave Preparation:

Place asparagus, tips toward the center, on a 12-inch round microwavable platter; sprinkle with 2 tablespoons water. Cover with vented plastic wrap and microwave on HIGH for 3 minutes, or until tender-crisp. Sprinkle peppers over the top. Recover and let stand for 1½ minutes. Proceed as above.

PYRAMID EQUIVALENT (SALAD ONLY): ½ FRUIT, 1½ VEGETABLES

Nutritional Analysis per Portion (salad and vinaigrette)

calories 90 ▲ carbohydrate 13 grams ▲ protein 4 grams ▲ fat 4 grams
sodium 4 milligrams ▲ cholesterol 0 milligrams

▲▲

ITALIAN BREAD SALAD

(PANZANELLA)

MAKES 4 PORTIONS

Panzanella, a rustic Italian dish, has as many variations as it has chefs. This one is especially good in summer when ripe, juicy tomatoes abound.

A hearty whole-grain or sourdough bread is a good choice.

8 ounces stale 1-inch bread cubes (about 4 cups)
3 large ripe tomatoes, coarsely chopped (about 1 pound)
$\frac{1}{2}$ cup sliced celery
$\frac{1}{2}$ cup thinly sliced red onion
2 tablespoons capers, drained
2 garlic cloves, minced
5 large basil leaves, shredded
3 sage leaves, chopped fine
3 tablespoons balsamic vinegar
2 tablespoons extra-virgin olive oil
Freshly ground pepper to taste

Briefly moisten the bread with cold water; squeeze out excess moisture.
In a large bowl, combine all the ingredients and toss well to combine.
Let the salad stand for about 10 minutes. Serve at room temperature.

PYRAMID EQUIVALENT: 2 BREADS, 2 VEGETABLES

Nutritional Analysis per Portion

calories 239 ▲ carbohydrate 34 grams ▲ protein 8 grams ▲ fat 9 grams
sodium 505 milligrams ▲ cholesterol 0 milligrams

▲▲

SPINACH, CITRUS, AND GOAT CHEESE SALAD

MAKES 4 PORTIONS

If you're looking for a beta carotene fix and want a simple and stylish salad, this is just the ticket. Spinach is a powerhouse of nutrition: it's rich in beta carotene, iron, and vitamin A. Here it is complemented by the sweetness and bright color of the mandarin oranges and by crumbly goat cheese.

4 cups fresh spinach, washed and trimmed (about 8 ounces)
1 cup thinly sliced mushrooms (about 6 large)
1 11-ounce can mandarin orange sections, drained
$1/4$ cup orange juice
1 tablespoon fresh lemon juice
2 teaspoons EACH vegetable oil and honey
$1/8$ teaspoon freshly ground black pepper
3 ounces dry goat cheese or feta cheese, crumbled (about $1/2$ cup)

Tear spinach into bite-size pieces and place in a large salad bowl. Add mushrooms and orange sections.

In a small bowl whisk together the remaining ingredients, except the cheese. Pour over the salad, and toss well to combine.

Distribute the mixture among four chilled salad plates. Sprinkle some of the goat cheese over each.

PYRAMID EQUIVALENT: 1 $1/2$ VEGETABLES, $1/2$ FRUIT, $1/2$ MILK

Nutritional Analysis per Portion

calories 199 ▲ carbohydrate 21 grams ▲ protein 9 grams ▲ fat 10 grams
sodium 124 milligrams ▲ cholesterol 22 milligrams

▲▲

SESAME-DRESSED FIELD GREENS WITH APPLES AND WATER CHESTNUTS

MAKES 4 PORTIONS

Use any of your favorite field greens, or try a mix of Bibb and Romaine lettuces with some spinach if you tend toward the less exotic. Look for Gala apples when they're available, September through December. This variety is similar to a Golden

Delicious, but with a touch of tartness that adds just the right lilt to this salad. The blushed skin is so attractive, I don't bother peeling these beauties. For some reason even the experts couldn't explain to me, Gala apples don't oxidize (turn brown) as quickly as other varieties, so if you use them this salad can be assembled in up to 4 hours in advance (without the dressing).

> 6 cups mixed field greens, washed thoroughly and dried
> 1 8-ounce can low-sodium sliced water chestnuts, drained
> 1 medium Gala or Golden Delicious apple (about 6 ounces), cored and cut
>   into $\frac{1}{2}$-inch dice
> $\frac{1}{3}$ cup Sesame Dressing (page 124)

In a large bowl toss all ingredients thoroughly.

PYRAMID EQUIVALENT (SALAD ONLY): $\frac{1}{4}$ FRUIT, 2 VEGETABLES

Nutritional Analysis per Portion (salad and dressing)

calories 113 ▲ carbohydrate 19 grams ▲ protein 9 grams ▲ fat 10 grams
sodium 55 milligrams ▲ cholesterol 0 milligrams

▲▲

LEMONY DILL DRESSING

MAKES ABOUT $\frac{1}{2}$ CUP

Pour this tart dressing over grain salads. It's especially nice with barley or lentils, and it adds a tangy accent to chicken or seafood salads.

> $\frac{1}{4}$ cup fresh lemon juice
> 2 tablespoons water
> 1 tablespoon canola oil
> 1 teaspoon Dijon mustard
> 1 tablespoon chopped fresh dill
> Dash Tabasco sauce

In a small bowl whisk all ingredients together until blended, or combine in a blender until smooth.

▲▲

CILANTRO-LIME DRESSING

MAKES ABOUT ¾ CUP

A hint of ground cumin gives this piquant dressing a smoky, southwestern touch. It's a good partner for a pasta salad, and it also goes well with beans and grains.

¼ cup EACH chicken broth (see page 40) and fresh lime juice
2 tablespoons EACH olive oil and water
¼ cup chopped fresh cilantro
1 teaspoon grated lime peel (green part only)
¾ teaspoon EACH ground cumin and dry mustard
Salt and pepper to taste

In a small bowl whisk all ingredients together until blended, or combine in a blender until smooth.

▲▲▲

HONEY-DIJON DRESSING

MAKES ABOUT ½ CUP

Chicken (or vegetable) broth helps to replace some of the oil here. Use an extra-virgin olive oil, which has a fuller, "fruitier" flavor than regular olive oil, and you won't miss the usual amount one bit.

¼ cup white wine vinegar
3 tablespoons chicken broth (see page 40)
2 teaspoons EACH extra-virgin olive oil and Dijon mustard
1 ½ teaspoons honey
1 or 2 large garlic cloves, pressed
¼ teaspoon freshly ground black pepper

In a small bowl whisk all ingredients together until blended, or combine in a blender until smooth.

Nutritional Analysis per Tablespoon

calories 19 ▲ carbohydrate 2 grams ▲ protein 0 grams ▲ fat 1 gram
sodium 39 milligrams ▲ cholesterol 0 milligrams

▲▲▲

SESAME DRESSING

MAKES ABOUT ½ CUP

Fresh ginger perks up a dressing. This one is nice with mixed greens, or toss it with noodles and shredded vegetables for an Oriental touch.

3 tablespoons cider vinegar
2 tablespoons white wine vinegar
I tablespoon plus I teaspoon vegetable oil
I tablespoon orange juice
I teaspoon finely chopped fresh ginger, or to taste
Dash ground red pepper
2 teaspoons toasted sesame seeds

Combine all ingredients, except sesame seeds, and whisk together until blended, or combine in a blender until smooth. Add sesame seeds and serve, or cover and store in refrigerator.

Nutritional Analysis per Tablespoon

calories 26 ▲ carbohydrate I gram ▲ protein 0 grams ▲ fat 3 grams
sodium 0 milligrams ▲ cholesterol 0 milligrams

▲▲▲

APRICOT VINAIGRETTE

MAKES ABOUT ½ CUP

Feel free to add your favorite chopped herbs—basil, thyme, cilantro, etc.—to this easy dressing. It stores well in the refrigerator for about 2 weeks. You may want to double the recipe and keep lots on hand.

$1/3$ cup apricot nectar
1 tablespoon EACH canola oil and cider vinegar
1 teaspoon fresh lime juice
$1/4$ teaspoon EACH dry mustard and ground coriander
Dash Tabasco sauce

In a small bowl whisk all ingredients together until blended, or combine in a blender until smooth.

Nutritional Analysis per Tablespoon

calories 22 ▲ carbohydrate 2 grams ▲ protein 0 grams ▲ fat 2 grams
sodium 1 milligram ▲ cholesterol 0 milligrams

▲▲

SLIMMING DOWN SALAD DRESSINGS

Keep the following tricks in mind for salads that are nutritious and low in fat:

▲ Increase herbs and spices in dressings. Include tarragon, dill, chervil, curry and chili powders, oregano, marjoram, and mint, in addition to parsley, basil, and thyme.

▲ Use fresh and canned juices to add new flavors. Canned nectars like apricot, mango, and pear nectar add texture and thickness in addition to flavor.

▲ Try nonfat yogurt and reduced-calorie mayonnaise to replace just over half the amount of sour cream and/or regular mayonnaise called for in most recipes.

▲ Replace some of the customary oil with vegetable or chicken broth to maintain the flavor of dressings.

▲ Prepare dressings in a blender and add a touch of prepared or dry mustard to give them extra body.

▲ Cook a half cup of broth or juice, with a teaspoon of cornstarch whisked into it, in a small saucepan, over medium heat, until it just comes to a boil; stir for 30 seconds and cool. Add vinegar and flavorings. The cooked cornstarch makes a smoother, thicker dressing.

▲▲

▲▲

CREAMY TARRAGON DRESSING

MAKES ABOUT I CUP

You'll hardly miss the fat in this creamy yogurt dressing. I love it tossed with fresh vegetables, and the tarragon is especially good with chicken or smoked turkey.

 $^1\!/_2$ cup EACH nonfat plain yogurt and reduced-calorie mayonnaise
 I tablespoon chopped fresh tarragon or I $^1\!/_2$ teaspoons dried, crumbled
 $^1\!/_4$ teaspoon freshly ground black pepper

In a small bowl whisk all ingredients together until blended, or combine in a blender until smooth.

Nutritional Analysis per Tablespoon

calories 25 ▲ carbohydrate I gram ▲ protein I gram ▲ fat 2 grams
sodium 46 milligrams ▲ cholesterol 3 milligrams

▲▲

EASY TOMATO SAUCE

MAKES 5 CUPS

A number of other ingredients can be added to this sauce, including fennel, rosemary, parsley, thyme, or even some fresh mint. This one goes with just about anything and freezes well so you can always have it on hand.

1 tablespoon EACH extra-virgin olive oil and water
1 cup finely chopped onion
3 garlic cloves, minced
6 cups coarsely chopped ripe tomatoes (about 2 pounds)
3 tablespoons chopped fresh basil
1/2 teaspoon sugar
Pinch salt and dried red pepper flakes
1 tablespoon balsamic vinegar, optional

In a large saucepan heat oil over medium-high heat; add onion and cook for 3 minutes. Add garlic and cook 2 minutes longer; add remaining ingredients. Reduce heat to low and cook, stirring occasionally, for about 20 minutes, or until sauce has thickened.

PYRAMID EQUIVALENT (PER CUP): 2 VEGETABLES

Nutritional Analysis per Cup

calories 80 ▲ carbohydrate 13 grams ▲ protein 2 grams ▲ fat 3 grams
sodium 44 milligrams ▲ cholesterol 0 milligrams

▲▲

QUICK TOMATO SAUCE

MAKES ABOUT 5 CUPS

When you're really in a hurry, or don't have fresh ingredients on hand, this makes a very nice sauce. It, too, freezes well. I like to use Eden brand canned tomatoes for several reasons: they're organic, have no added salt, and the cans are enamel-lined and lead-free, so there's no bitter taste. They are sold in most health food stores and have made their way into many local supermarkets.

3 15-ounce cans no-salt-added crushed tomatoes (about 6 cups)
2 teaspoons garlic paste concentrate, or to taste, or 2 to 3 garlic cloves,
    minced
1 1/2 teaspoons dried basil, crumbled
1 teaspoon dried oregano, crumbled
Pinch salt and dried pepper flakes
1 tablespoon balsamic vinegar, optional

In a large saucepan combine all the ingredients, and bring to a boil. Reduce heat to low and simmer, stirring occasionally, for about 20 minutes.

PYRAMID EQUIVALENT (PER CUP): 2 VEGETABLES

Nutritional Analysis per Cup

calories 55 ▲ carbohydrate 12 grams ▲ protein 3 grams ▲ fat 1 gram
sodium 60 milligrams ▲ cholesterol 0 milligrams

▲▲

GRANNY'S APPLESAUCE

MAKES 4 PORTIONS

Leaving the skin on apples gives a rosy hue to homemade applesauce. But I was dazzled when a friend's grandmother, Evelyn Weiner, made the loveliest and freshest tasting applesauce I ever sampled. Her secret ingredient is plums. I think you'll agree this applesauce is perfect with no added sugar.

    3 pounds Cortland, Winesap, or Jonathan apples, cored and quartered
        (about 8 medium)
    1 pound Santa Rosa plums, pitted and quartered (about 4 medium)
    2/3 cup water
    1 tablespoon lemon juice
    1 cinnamon stick, 3 inches long
    3 allspice berries, optional

In a large saucepan, combine all ingredients. Bring to a boil over high heat. Reduce heat and simmer, stirring occasionally, for 20 to 25 minutes, or until fruit has softened. Put the fruit, with its juices, through a food mill or press through a sieve.

PYRAMID EQUIVALENT: 3 FRUITS

Nutritional Analysis per Portion

calories 224 ▲ carbohydrate 57 grams ▲ protein 1 gram ▲ fat 2 grams
sodium 0 milligrams ▲ cholesterol 0 milligrams

▲▲

BLUEBERRY SAUCE

MAKES 2 CUPS

This is a simple, fruity, and fat-free sauce that is sublime over ice cream, frozen yogurt, Angel Food Cake (page 185), or Plum Good Bread Pudding (page 188). It was developed quite by accident when I was giving a microwave class at Bristol Farms Cook 'n Things in Los Angeles. I had planned to demonstrate a cranberry sauce recipe; but when cranberries were not available at the last minute, my able assistant, David Forstel, scouted out some fresh blueberries instead. Here's the result.

3 cups fresh blueberries, rinsed and drained
3 tablespoons granulated or turbinado sugar*
1/4 cup Myers's dark rum
1/4 teaspoon vanilla

In a 4-cup glass measure or 1-quart microwave casserole combine all ingredients. Microwave on HIGH for 4 to 6 minutes, or until blueberries start to pop and sauce begins to thicken. Stir once during cooking.

* Turbinado, a less refined sugar, is available at health food stores.

Let stand to cool slightly. Serve warm, or store in a tightly covered container in the refrigerator.

Stovetop Preparation:

In a 1-quart nonmetallic saucepan, combine all ingredients. Heat over medium-high heat until just boiling; reduce heat and simmer, stirring occasionally, for about 10 minutes, until blueberries start to pop and sauce begins to thicken. Proceed as directed above.

PYRAMID EQUIVALENT (PER $1/4$ CUP): $1/2$ FRUIT

Nutritional Analysis per $1/4$ Cup

calories 65 ▲ carbohydrate 12 grams ▲ protein 0 grams ▲ fat 0 grams
sodium 3 milligrams ▲ cholesterol 0 milligrams

▲▲

CHICKEN BROTH (STOCK)

MAKES ABOUT 3 QUARTS

Making broth (stock) from scratch is simple, and the results are so gratifying. It's a pleasure to reach in the freezer and pull some out whenever you need it.

Use chicken parts from a roaster, since these older birds are more flavorful. This is also the time to use the cooked carcass from the Toreador Chicken (page 145). There's no added salt here, so the stock is almost sodium-free and after you have removed the fat it is almost fat-free. Use the meat for salads, pasta, or grain dishes; it'll be moist, tender, and flavorful.

1 chicken carcass with some meat left on or 3 to 4 pounds roaster parts
4 quarts water
2 celery stalks with leaves, chopped coarse
2 carrots, peeled and chopped coarse
1 large onion, peeled and quartered
12 parsley sprigs
4 whole black peppercorns
2 bay leaves
1 teaspoon dried thyme leaves, crumbled

In a stockpot combine all the ingredients and add enough water to cover chicken by about an inch. Cover and bring to a boil; reduce heat and simmer for 2 hours. Skim stock occasionally with a large spoon to remove any fat and foam.

Remove carcass (or chicken parts) from pot. Cut away meat from bones and reserve for another use; discard fat and bones.

Strain remaining stock through a strainer or colander lined with cheesecloth, and chill overnight. With a spoon, lift hardened fat off the top of stock and discard.

Transfer the stock to smaller containers. Store in the refrigerator for about 2 weeks or in the freezer for several months.

Pressure Cooker Preparation:

In an 8-quart pressure cooker heat oil and cook vegetables; then add ingredients as directed above. Lock the lid in place and cook on high pressure for 15 minutes; let pressure drop on its own. Proceed as above. (Note: A 4- or 6-quart cooker may be used; reduce vegetables and water so cooker is no more than three-quarters full. Use the same timing.)

Nutritional Analysis per Cup

calories 39 ▲ carbohydrate 3 grams ▲ protein 3 grams ▲ fat 2 grams
sodium 65 milligrams ▲ cholesterol 0 milligrams

VEGETABLE BROTH (STOCK)

MAKES ABOUT 3 ½ QUARTS

Don't be daunted by the list of ingredients here. Once the ingredients are assembled they all go right into the pot; there are no complicated steps after that. This broth (stock) is rich and flavorful: it's meant to be that way so when you use it in other recipes you can leave out the fat and never miss it.

2 tablespoons vegetable oil
4 medium leeks thoroughly rinsed and sliced (green tops included)
3 celery stalks, with leaves, chopped
3 medium carrots, peeled and chopped coarse
2 large garlic cloves
10–12 sprigs parsley
6 black peppercorns
6 juniper berries
2 bay leaves
¾ teaspoon dried thyme, crumbled
Generous pinch crushed red pepper
4 quarts water
2 tablespoons balsamic vinegar

In a stockpot heat the oil. Add the leeks, celery, carrots, and garlic. Cook for 5 minutes, or until the leeks are just translucent, stirring occasionally.

Add the remaining ingredients, except the vinegar. Bring to a boil and reduce heat to low. Cover partially and simmer for 2 hours; stir in the vinegar.

Pour the stock through a strainer or colander lined with cheesecloth, pressing out excess liquid with the back of a spoon.

Transfer the stock to smaller containers. Store in the refrigerator for about 2 weeks, or in the freezer for several months.

In an 8-quart pressure cooker heat oil and cook vegetables, and add ingredients as directed above. Lock the lid in place, and cook on high pressure for 10 minutes; let pressure drop on its own. Proceed as above. (Note: A 4- or 6-quart cooker may be used; reduce vegetables and water so cooker is no more than three-quarters full. Use same timing.)

Nutritional Analysis per Cup

calories 24 ▲ carbohydrate 2 grams ▲ protein 0 grams ▲ fat 2 grams
sodium 6 milligrams ▲ cholesterol 0 milligrams

▲▲▲

MAIN COURSES

ROASTED COD WITH PEPPERS, ONIONS, AND NEW POTATOES

STEAMED CATFISH THAI-STYLE

GINGER-STEAMED FISH

LINGUINE WITH SHRIMP AND BROCCOLI

TURKEY POT AU FEU

MIXED BEANS AND CHICKEN STEW

TOREADOR CHICKEN

THREE-WAY ROAST CHICKEN

WHOLE-GRAIN MEAT LOAF

GRILLED BANGKOK BEEF SALAD

SIZZLING PORK POCKETS

BROCHETTES OF VENISON WITH ROSEMARY-JUNIPER SAUCE

VENISON AND RED BEAN CHILI

GREEK RABBIT STEW

LAMB SALAD WITH GREEN BEANS

PENNE WITH BEANS AND GREENS

NO-FAT/NO-SWEAT LASAGNA WITH SPINACH AND LENTILS

SAFFRON-SCENTED RISOTTO WITH PORTOBELLO MUSHROOMS

BLUSHING PINK RISOTTO WITH BAROLO WINE

BLACK BEAN CHILI WITH RED PEPPERS AND CORN

VEGETARIAN STIR-FRY HUNAN-STYLE

VEGETABLE LO MEIN

PAD THAI

CAJUN LENTIL CAKES

▲▲▲

The recommendation of 5 to 7 ounces of protein for an entire day is probably far below what most people are currently consuming. Americans have become accustomed to estimate at least 8 ounces of roast chicken per person and to buy steaks large enough so that each guest has 12 to 14 ounces on his or her plate.

Eating more grains, more fruit and vegetables, more fiber, less protein, and less fat means redirecting portion sizes and reevaluating the kinds of foods we choose to eat on a regular basis. It may take a little time to retrain your thinking about eating 3 ounces of protein (or less) in one meal, so it will be easier if the transition is a gradual one. (Of course you could choose to have the full 5 or 7 ounces at one meal and fill in with fruits, vegetables, pasta, and salads at the others.)

What I've done in the following recipes is to help you through that transition by keeping the look of your plate familiar in the recipes at the beginning of the chapter, where protein is still the center of attraction, as in Roasted Cod with Peppers, Onions, and New Potatoes or Brochettes of Venison with Rosemary-Juniper Sauce. Linguine with Shrimp and Broccoli and Mixed Beans and Chicken Stew are dishes with more vegetables and complex carbohydrates and less protein; and finally, recipes like Vegetable Lo Mein and Saffron-scented Risotto with Portobello Mushrooms are completely meatless, for those who are vegetarians or who want to work in a few meatless meals now and then.

In all of the recipes there is a distinct emphasis on replacing fat with flavor. Toreador Chicken, for example, is prepared on a vertical roaster so the maximum amount of fat drains off during cooking; a mustard-tarragon mixture is tucked under the skin to enhance the natural flavor of the chicken. A tad of chili oil and some fresh ginger bring up the flavors of Vegetarian Stir-Fry Hunan-Style. Penne with Beans and Greens, seasoned with thyme, crushed red pepper flakes, and grated Parmesan cheese, is hearty and delicious. I hope you'll try both of the risottos, and I especially hope you'll consider getting a pressure cooker if you don't already own one. It will produce the likes of a hand-stirred risotto, which usually takes up to half an hour, in just five minutes—without any stirring. If you're looking for quick and easy, look at the No-Fat/No-Sweat Lasagna, in which you layer all the ingredients *without* cooking the noodles first. This is a recipe where nonfat cheeses don't dry out (as they are prone to do). They stay moist because of the sauce that surrounds them.

▲▲

ROASTED COD WITH PEPPERS, ONIONS, AND NEW POTATOES

MAKES 4 PORTIONS

Cod is a delicate, mild-tasting fish with a low fat content. Roasting sweet bell peppers, onions, and red potatoes right in the same pan makes this an easy and colorful dish. Scrod, haddock, or hake are almost as low in fat and calories as cod, if you're looking for a stand-in.

> 3 cups red and yellow bell peppers, seeded and cut into 2 × ½-inch strips
> 1 cup thinly sliced onion
> 1¼ pounds small red (new) potatoes, scrubbed and cut into ½-inch
>   wedges
> 1 tablespoon plus 1 teaspoon extra-virgin olive oil
> 1½ teaspoons dried thyme leaves, crumbled
> ½ teaspoon dried marjoram leaves, crumbled
> 1¼ pounds cod
> 2 tablespoons balsamic vinegar, or to taste
> Salt and freshly ground pepper to taste

Preheat oven to 425° F.

In a large roasting pan toss peppers, onion, potatoes, 1 tablespoon oil, 1 teaspoon thyme, and marjoram until vegetables are lightly coated with oil. Bake for 20 minutes, stirring twice (add a bit of water if necessary).

Push vegetables to sides of the pan; place the cod, skin side down, in the center. Rub remaining oil over the top and sprinkle with remaining thyme. Bake for about 15 minutes, or until fish flakes easily with a fork.

Place fish on a heated platter. Pour vinegar over vegetables; add salt and pepper to taste, and stir to combine (add additional vinegar or a bit of water, if desired). Spoon over fish and serve.

PYRAMID EQUIVALENT: 1 1/2 VEGETABLES, 3 3/4 OUNCES COOKED FISH

Nutritional Analysis per Portion

calories 309 ▲ carbohydrate 34 grams ▲ protein 29 grams ▲ fat 6 grams
sodium 91 milligrams ▲ cholesterol 61 milligrams

▲▲

STEAMED CATFISH THAI-STYLE

MAKES 4 PORTIONS

Catfish is very popular in Thailand. It's also very low in fat. This spicy version contains no added fat so it's about as low-cal as you can get. Serve it on a bed of steamed spinach for an attractive presentation.

2 tablespoons orange juice
1 1/2 tablespoons fish sauce (nam pla)*
1/4 cup chopped cilantro, divided
1 scallion (green onion), including about 1 inch of the green top, sliced thin
1/4 teaspoon paprika
1/8 teaspoon ground red pepper
1 pound catfish fillets

* Available at Asian markets or in the ethnic foods section in some supermarkets.

In a skillet large enough to hold the catfish, combine all ingredients except 2 tablespoons of the cilantro and the catfish. Bring to a boil, and cook for 1 minute.

Place the catfish in the pan in a single layer. Cover and cook over medium heat for 5 minutes, or until the fish is just done.

Transfer the fish to a heated platter. Pour the juices over the top and garnish with remaining cilantro.

PYRAMID EQUIVALENT: 3 OUNCES COOKED FISH

Nutritional Analysis per Portion

calories 165 ▲ carbohydrate 2 grams ▲ protein 18 grams ▲ fat 9 grams
sodium 38 milligrams ▲ cholesterol 37 milligrams

▲▲

GINGER-STEAMED FISH

MAKES 4 PORTIONS

This dish is remarkably easy to prepare and impressive to serve. You can enhance the presentation by topping the fish with thinly sliced tomatoes or onions and surrounding it with shredded carrot or zucchini or sliced mushrooms just before steaming. Use white wine, vegetable stock, or fish stock, or add herbs and peppercorns to the steaming liquid as other variations.

1 whole sea bass, rock cod, or red snapper, scaled and cleaned (about 2
    pounds) with head and tail left on (if steamer space permits)
1 2-inch piece ginger, peeled and cut into 4 slices
3 scallions (green onions), trimmed
2 tablespoons rice vinegar or sherry
2 tablespoons low-sodium soy sauce

Rinse the fish with cold water and pat dry; make three light slashes on each side. Cut one of the scallions into thin shreds; set aside. Put the ginger slices and the two remaining scallions inside the fish.

Place fish on a plate that will fit on a steamer rack*; rub 1 tablespoon of the vinegar and 1 tablespoon of the soy sauce over the fish.

Add about 2 inches of water (or stock and seasonings as suggested above) to the steamer; bring to a boil. Place the plate on rack (cut fish in half if necessary to fit in steamer; reassemble to serve). Cover the steamer tightly and steam for about 15 minutes, or until fish looks just opaque. Scatter the reserved scallions over the top; sprinkle the remaining tablespoon of rice vinegar and tablespoon of soy sauce over the fish. Serve immediately, spooning some of the accumulated juices over the top of each portion.

* An authentic Chinese bamboo steamer is quite inexpensive to buy, but you can use a wok, which probably has its own steamer rack; or you can place two wooden chopsticks about 2 inches apart inside the wok and lay a heatproof plate on top. A collapsible vegetable steamer in a large, deep skillet holds a plate well too.

PYRAMID EQUIVALENT: 3 OUNCES COOKED FISH

Nutritional Analysis per Portion

calories 96 ▲ carbohydrate 2 grams ▲ protein 17 grams ▲ fat 2 grams
sodium 363 milligrams ▲ cholesterol 36 milligrams

▲▲

LINGUINE WITH SHRIMP AND BROCCOLI

MAKES 4 PORTIONS

Shrimp and other once-forbidden shellfish are back on the "acceptable" list for just about everyone. These crustaceans haven't changed, but what we know about them has: their cholesterol is lower than was once thought.

³/₄ cup chicken broth (see page 40)

1 tablespoon extra-virgin olive oil

3 cups broccoli florets (about 6 ounces)

1 cup chopped tomato

¹/₄ cup chopped oil-cured olives

¹/₄ teaspoon crushed red pepper, or to taste

³/₄ pound medium shrimp, cleaned and deveined

¹/₂ pound linguine, cooked

In a large skillet bring the broth and oil to a boil; add broccoli. Cover and reduce heat to medium-low. Cook for 3 minutes, or until the broccoli is tender-crisp. Stir in the tomato, olives, pepper, and shrimp. Cook for 3 minutes, or until the shrimp turns pink and is done. Place linguine in a large serving bowl. Pour the broccoli-shrimp mixture over the top. Serve immediately.

PYRAMID EQUIVALENT: 2 BREADS,
1¹/₄ VEGETABLES, 3 OUNCES COOKED FISH

Nutritional Analysis per Portion

calories 372 ▲ carbohydrate 48 grams ▲ protein 24 grams ▲ fat 9 grams
sodium 425 milligrams ▲ cholesterol 105 milligrams

▲▲

TURKEY POT AU FEU

MAKES 4 PORTIONS

A classic French dish, this pot au feu gets a whole new look when boneless turkey breast stands in for the beef that is traditionally used. Some crusty sourdough bread, a salad, and dried California figs make this an easy-as-can-be meal.

4 cups chicken broth (see page 40)
6 sprigs fresh parsley
6 whole black peppercorns
4 whole cloves or allspice berries
1 bay leaf
1 teaspoon dried thyme
1 1/4 pounds fresh skinless, boneless turkey breast
2 cups butternut squash, peeled and cut into 1-inch cubes
1 cup thinly sliced carrot
1 cup thinly sliced onion
2 leeks, well rinsed and cut into 1-inch pieces

In a large saucepan or Dutch oven, bring chicken broth to a boil. Make a bouquet garni: In a 4-inch square of cheesecloth, place parsley, peppercorns, cloves, bay leaf, and thyme. Tie cheesecloth closed to form bag; place in broth. Reduce heat to low, and simmer for 15 minutes. Add remaining ingredients. Cover partially and bring just to a boil over high heat. Reduce heat and simmer pot au feu for 30 minutes, or until turkey is cooked through; turn turkey breast over once during cooking. Discard bouquet garni. Remove meat; slice thin and place in individual soup bowls. Spoon vegetables and broth over turkey.

PYRAMID EQUIVALENT: 2 VEGETABLES, 4 OUNCES COOKED POULTRY

Nutritional Analysis per Portion

calories 265 ▲ carbohydrate 20 grams ▲ protein 39 grams ▲ fat 3 grams
sodium 143 milligrams ▲ cholesterol 88 milligrams

▲▲

MIXED BEANS AND CHICKEN STEW

MAKES 4 PORTIONS

Here's an ideal Pyramid entrée: two kinds of beans, fresh vegetables, chunks of chicken, all in a heart-warming dish. I like to use thighs for their fuller flavor; you can buy them already skinned and boned. You could also use your slow cooker (Crock-Pot) here. Set it on HIGH and cook all the ingredients for 2 to 3 hours.

- 1 pound skinless, boneless chicken thighs
- 2 teaspoons extra-virgin olive oil
- 1 cup chopped onion
- 2 large garlic cloves, minced
- 1 teaspoon dried basil, crumbled
- 1/2 teaspoon EACH rosemary, oregano, and thyme
- 3/4 cup beef broth or water
- 2 cups EACH cooked cannellini and red kidney beans or canned beans, rinsed and drained
- 6 Italian plum tomatoes, chopped coarse
- 2 cups sliced carrots
- 1 large bay leaf
- 1/2 teaspoon freshly ground black pepper

Trim and discard visible fat from chicken thighs; cut thighs into 2-inch pieces. In a Dutch oven or large enamel casserole heat oil over medium-high heat. Add chicken and onion and cook for 5 minutes, or until brown on all sides. Add remaining ingredients. Reduce heat; cover and simmer for about 40 minutes, or until chicken is tender and cooked through.

Nutritional Analysis per Portion

calories 441 ▲ carbohydrate 54 grams ▲ protein 39 grams ▲ fat 8 grams
sodium 129 milligrams ▲ cholesterol 94 milligrams

▲▲

TOREADOR CHICKEN

MAKES 4 PORTIONS AND ABOUT 18 OUNCES
FOR LEFTOVER USE

I never really paid attention to the vertical chicken roasters I saw in cookware stores until I realized that they cut cooking time 30 to 40 percent, require less salt because birds are moister and juicer, and drain off more fat because of the vertical position. Carving and cleanup are a snap. This recipe got its name because my friend Cristina thinks that the chicken perched on the roaster looks like a toreador.

This recipe uses a simple blend of mustard, paprika, and tarragon. The 4½-pound roaster will yield about 3 ounces of cooked meat (without skin and bone) per person for four people and about 18 ounces left over for use in salads, casseroles, and rice or pasta dishes. Here's your chance to save the carcass and cook up some Chicken Stock (page 131).

3 tablespoons Dijon mustard
¾ teaspoon dried tarragon leaves, crushed
½ teaspoon paprika
¼ teaspoon freshly ground black pepper
1 4½-pound roaster
½ cup water

Preheat oven to 450° F.

In a small bowl combine all the ingredients except the chicken and water; set aside.

Place the roaster on its back and slip your forefingers under the skin at the neck opening on each side of the breast. Continue to work your fingers under the skin down the sides of the bird to form a pocket. Insert about ½ of the mustard mixture under the skin on each side; press the skin lightly to spread the mixture.

Place bird firmly on the roaster and set it in a 9-inch cake pan; pour in the water. Bake for 15 minutes; reduce oven temperature to 400° F and cook for about 1 hour (allow 12 to 15 minutes per pound). Let stand 5 minutes before carving.

Variations

Other combinations for "under the skin" flavorings can include:

> sliced fruits: oranges, apples, pineapple
> barbecue sauce
> flavored mustard
> Mexican salsa

PYRAMID EQUIVALENT: 3 OUNCES COOKED POULTRY
PER SERVING, 18 OUNCES COOKED POULTRY FOR LEFTOVER USE

Nutritional Analysis per Portion

calories 148 ▲ carbohydrate 1 gram ▲ protein 21 grams ▲ fat 6 grams
sodium 199 milligrams ▲ cholesterol 64 milligrams

▲▲

THREE-WAY ROAST CHICKEN

MAKES 6 PORTIONS AND ABOUT 22 OUNCES
FOR LEFTOVER USE

Many microwave owners spent lots of money for a "combination oven." That means they also have the convenience of a convection oven. Few people I know use this option, but to me it's a fine way to roast chicken. To speed things up, many ovens have a "mix" cycle that combines microwave cooking with the convection process. Whether you have a conventional, combination, or convection oven, here's a delicious and basic roast chicken anyone can make.

    1 6-pound roaster
    1 celery rib, cut in 3 pieces
    1 carrot, cut in 3 pieces
    1 small onion, halved
    2 sprigs fresh rosemary or thyme, optional

Conventional Preparation:

Preheat oven to 350° F.

Place roaster on a rack in a roasting pan; place vegetables inside chicken cavity. Roast chicken for about 2 hours, or until juices no longer run pink when thigh is pricked or a meat thermometer inserted in the thickest part of the inner thigh registers 180° F.

Convection Oven Preparation:

Preheat oven to 350° F.

Place roaster on a rack in a roasting pan; place vegetables inside chicken cavity. Roast chicken for about 1¾ hours, or until juices no longer run pink when thigh is pricked or a meat thermometer inserted in the thickest part of the inner thigh registers 180° F.

Microwave/Convection Mix:

Place roaster on a rack in a roasting pan; place vegetables inside chicken cavity. Roast chicken on HIGH/MIX for about 1 hour, or until juices no longer run pink when thigh is pricked or a meat thermometer inserted in the thickest part of the inner thigh registers 180° F.

PYRAMID EQUIVALENT: 3 OUNCES COOKED POULTRY
PER SERVING, 22 OUNCES COOKED POULTRY FOR LEFTOVER USE

Nutritional Analysis per Portion

calories 142 ▲ carbohydrate 0 grams ▲ protein 21 grams ▲ fat 6 grams
sodium 64 milligrams ▲ cholesterol 64 milligrams

▲▲▲

WHOLE-GRAIN MEAT LOAF

MAKES 6 PORTIONS

Extra-lean ground beef is a good way to keep the nutritional benefits of beef in your diet. It contains less than half the fat of regular ground beef, and almost half the fat and a third fewer calories compared to ground chicken and ground turkey. Instead of striking meat loaf off the menu, try this one, which uses bulgur instead of breadcrumbs. You'll get more fiber and flavor that way.

1 1/4 cups no-salt-added stewed tomatoes
1 pound extra-lean ground beef
4 egg whites, lightly beaten
1/2 cup medium bulgur
1/2 cup EACH chopped onion and green bell pepper
1/2 teaspoon EACH dried thyme and freshly ground black pepper

Preheat oven to 350° F.

Set aside about 1/3 cup of tomato pieces without their juice.

In a large bowl combine the remaining ingredients; do not overmix. Spoon the mixture into an 8 × 4-inch loaf pan (reduce oven temperature to 325° F if using glass); smooth to make an even layer. Place the reserved tomato pieces over the top. Bake for 55 minutes, or until an instant-reading thermometer reads 160° F. Let the meat loaf rest, in the pan on a rack, for 10 minutes before slicing.

PYRAMID EQUIVALENT: 3/4 BREAD,
1 VEGETABLE, 2 OUNCES COOKED MEAT

Nutritional Analysis per Portion

calories 202 ▲ carbohydrate 14 grams ▲ protein 20 grams ▲ fat 8 grams
sodium 103 milligrams ▲ cholesterol 47 milligrams

▲▲

GRILLED BANGKOK BEEF SALAD

MAKES 4 PORTIONS

The way most Asians eat, you might say they've been wise to the Pyramid for centuries. Rice and noodles are the base of their diet, and fresh vegetables abound. Meat, chicken, and fish are added in much smaller amounts than we're accustomed to.

I can rarely visit an Asian restaurant without ordering this spicy salad. It is full of flavor, yet not a drop of oil is used in the dressing. Since grilling is one of America's favorite pastimes, this recipe is a nice move into ethnic cuisine. Note that nutritious spinach and Romaine leaves replace the iceberg lettuce generally used in this dish.

12 ounces lean top round (for London broil)*
1/4 cup fresh lime juice
1 tablespoon plus 1 teaspoon rice vinegar
2 teaspoons fish sauce (nam pla)** or low-sodium soy sauce
1/4 teaspoon crushed red pepper flakes, or to taste
3 cups EACH torn spinach and Romaine lettuce leaves
1 medium tomato, cored and cut into 6 wedges
1/2 cup EACH shredded carrot, bean sprouts, and thinly sliced red onion
1/4 cup chopped fresh mint leaves, for garnish

Preheat grill or broiler. Cook steak about 5 minutes on each side (for medium-rare), or until desired doneness. Set aside, or wrap in aluminum foil and refrigerate until ready to use; then slice across the grain into very thin slices.

In a large bowl combine the lime juice, rice vinegar, fish sauce or soy sauce, and pepper. Add the steak and remaining ingredients, except the red onion and mint; toss well. Transfer the salad to a large platter, and garnish with red onion and mint.

* Coleman Beef is one of several companies producing lean beef without using hormones or antibiotics. It is labeled by brand in the meat case at many supermarkets, or see page 226 for ordering information.
** Available at Asian markets or in the ethnic foods section in some supermarkets.

PYRAMID EQUIVALENT: 2¾ VEGETABLES, 2 OUNCES COOKED MEAT

Nutritional Analysis per Portion

calories 167 ▲ carbohydrate 10 grams ▲ protein 24 grams ▲ fat 4 grams
sodium 87 milligrams ▲ cholesterol 54 milligrams

▲▲

SIZZLING PORK POCKETS

MAKES 4 PORTIONS

Pork is 31 percent leaner and 29 percent lower in saturated fat than it was ten years ago; it's also a good source of thiamine, iron, and zinc. This easy stir-fry dish is practically a salad and sandwich all in one.

2 tablespoons EACH Dijon mustard, lemon juice, and chicken broth (see page 40)
2 garlic cloves, chopped fine
⅛ teaspoon freshly ground black pepper
12 ounces boneless pork loin, cut into thin strips
4 6-inch pita breads (about 2 ounces each)
2 cups chopped mixed lettuce
¼ cup Creamy Tarragon Dressing (page 127), optional

In a medium bowl combine the mustard, lemon juice, chicken broth, garlic, and pepper. Add the pork strips and toss to combine. Refrigerate and marinate for 15 to 20 minutes. Remove meat with a slotted spoon, and discard marinade.

Heat a large nonstick skillet or wok over medium-high heat. Stir-fry the pork for 5 minutes, or until done. Open pita breads to form a pocket and fill each with an even amount of lettuce and pork strips. Top with a tablespoon of Creamy Tarragon Dressing, if desired.

▲▲▲

BROCHETTES OF VENISON WITH ROSEMARY-JUNIPER SAUCE

MAKES 6 PORTIONS

Fire up the grill and get in step with easy game cookery. These kebabs can also be prepared in your broiler, or on the special hinges of a vertical chicken roaster (page 225). Game meat is naturally low in fat, and several kinds are now farm-raised, making it easier to buy all year long. Bill Bailey, a chef in New York City, developed this recipe. The sauce is light and full-flavored, without any added fat. Look for whole juniper berries in the spice section of your supermarket. I order venison from Broken Arrow Ranch in Texas (see page 226), and it's about the best I've eaten. Many local meat markets are now carrying venison or will order it for you.

2 cups orange juice
⅔ cup white wine vinegar
3 cups beef broth
2 tablespoons juniper berries, crushed
2 teaspoons fresh rosemary, chopped, or 1 teaspoon dried rosemary leaves
6 medium mushroom caps
2 pounds boneless hind leg of venison, cut into 2-inch cubes
1 red bell pepper, seeded and cored, cut into 6 strips
1 cup fresh or canned pineapple chunks
1 banana, cut into 6 chunks
6 10-inch bamboo skewers, soaked in water for 30 minutes
Salt and ground white pepper, to taste

In a small saucepan combine the orange juice, vinegar, and broth. Bring to a boil and cook over high heat 10 to 12 minutes or until syrupy, stirring occasionally. Add juniper berries and rosemary; cook over medium heat 5 minutes longer, stirring frequently. Strain the sauce and return to saucepan; keep warm.

Skewer ingredients to make 6 brochettes, starting with a mushroom cap and ending with a banana chunk, using several venison cubes in between. Place brochettes on a plate, and pour about half the sauce over the top. Refrigerate and let marinate for 20 to 30 minutes, turning occasionally. Sprinkle with salt and pepper to taste. Grill or broil 5 to 7 minutes, turning once during cooking. Place one brochette on each dinner plate and pour a small amount of the reserved sauce over each.

PYRAMID EQUIVALENT: $1/3$ FRUIT, $1/3$ VEGETABLE,
2 OUNCES COOKED MEAT

Nutritional Analysis per Portion

calories 257 ▲ carbohydrate 17 grams ▲ protein 37 grams ▲ fat 4 grams
sodium 389 milligrams ▲ cholesterol 129 milligrams

▲▲▲

VENISON AND RED BEAN CHILI

MAKES 6 PORTIONS

For those who just can't give up meat in their chili, venison is the perfect addition. Remember that it's low in fat.

Though the simplest chili always seems to include many ingredients, it's easy to put together. You can add a special touch to the recipe if you toast the cumin seeds in a toaster oven or in a dry skillet for about 3 minutes, then grind the spice in a blender or electric mill.

The Pyramid Equivalents here count the venison as protein and the beans as vegetables, though beans can also be an additional protein allowance if you've had a heavy salad day so far.

3 cups beef broth

1 pound ground venison

4 garlic cloves, minced

2½ cups sliced mushrooms (mix some field with porcini or Portobello, if desired)

2 cups chopped onions

¼ cup mild chili powder

1 tablespoon EACH ground cumin from toasted seeds, and dried oregano, crumbled

½ teaspoon EACH ground allspice and ground red pepper

2 14½-ounce cans no-salt-added stewed tomatoes (about 4 cups)

6 cups cooked small red chili beans or canned beans, rinsed and drained

1 tablespoon grated orange peel (orange part only)

Chopped cilantro, for garnish, optional

In a Dutch oven or large enamel casserole bring ⅓ cup of the broth to a boil. Add the meat and cook over medium-high heat for 5 minutes, stirring occasionally. Using a slotted spoon remove the meat, and set aside.

Add the garlic, mushrooms, onions, chili powder, cumin, oregano, allspice, and pepper; cook over high heat for 5 minutes longer, stirring occasionally. Add the remaining broth, the venison, tomatoes, and beans. Simmer, uncovered, for 45 minutes, stirring occasionally. Stir in the orange peel.

Ladle the chili into serving bowls and garnish with chopped cilantro, if desired.

PYRAMID EQUIVALENT: 3 VEGETABLES, 2 OUNCES COOKED MEAT

Nutritional Analysis per Portion

calories 365 ▲ carbohydrate 50 grams ▲ protein 33 grams ▲ fat 5 grams
sodium 640 milligrams ▲ cholesterol 64 milligrams

▲▲

GREEK RABBIT STEW

MAKES 6 PORTIONS

You can let Sunday dinner just about cook itself while you curl up on the couch with your favorite newspaper; then let the aroma of this fragrant stew call folks to the table. Greek cuisine, with its emphasis on vibrant flavors and healthful ingredients, has worked its way into today's changing tastes. Rabbit, with its lean profile, is low in calories, fat, and cholesterol, while high in protein, iron, and vitamin B_{12}.

Thanks to Florence Fabricant of the *New York Times* for adapting this recipe from Chris Veneris, a Greek chef who prepared the stew for a luncheon hosted by the Greek Food and Wine Institute. I have slightly refined the *Times* version for you. Rabbit is available in many specialty stores or can be ordered from Classic Country Rabbit Company in Oregon (page 226).

> 2 tablespoons extra-virgin olive oil
> 1 3-pound rabbit, cut into six large pieces (skinless chicken thighs may be substituted)
> 2 pounds pearl or small white onions, peeled (about 4 cups)*
> 4 large garlic cloves, peeled
> 15 whole black peppercorns
> 10 whole allspice berries
> 4 bay leaves
> 1 teaspoon ground cumin
> 1/2 cup dry red wine
> 1/3 cup red wine vinegar
> 6 medium tomatoes, cored and cut into chunks
> 1 orange, unpeeled, halved, and cut into thin slices
> 1/4 cup mint leaves, optional

In a large saucepan or Dutch oven heat the oil over high heat and cook the rabbit on both sides until golden brown; remove to a platter. Add the onions and garlic cloves,

* Frozen, whole small onions may also be used.

154

and cook, stirring occasionally, until lightly browned. Return the rabbit to the pan, and stir in the remaining ingredients, except the mint (if using).

Cover, bring to a boil, reduce heat, and simmer for 45 minutes, or until the rabbit and onions are tender. Using a slotted spoon, transfer the rabbit and vegetables to a heated platter; discard the bay leaves. Add the mint, if desired, to the sauce, and cook over high heat until slightly thickened. Remove the skin from the rabbit, and pour the sauce over the top.

PYRAMID EQUIVALENT: 2 ½ VEGETABLES, 5 OUNCES COOKED MEAT

Nutritional Analysis per Portion

calories 376 ▲ carbohydrate 25 grams ▲ protein 37 grams ▲ fat 15 grams
sodium 99 milligrams ▲ cholesterol 98 milligrams

▲▲

LAMB SALAD WITH GREEN BEANS

MAKES 4 PORTIONS

When I'm feeling extravagant, I sometimes use haricots verts, the ultra-thin French green beans. Though they are pricey, they add a nice touch. You can also trim regular green beans and place them lengthwise in the feed tube of a food processor for a very finely sliced bean.

12 ounces cooked lamb, cut into julienne strips (about 2 cups)
1 ½ cups cooked green beans or haricots verts
4 medium red (new) potatoes, cooked and quartered (about 12 ounces)
⅓ cup Honey-Dijon Dressing (page 124)
3 tablespoons chopped fresh mint
3 cups shredded Bibb or red leaf lettuce

155

In a medium bowl toss together all the ingredients except the lettuces. Cover and set aside for 30 minutes; or chill until ready to serve.

Distribute the lettuces among four plates. Toss the lamb mixture again, and place an equal amount on top of the greens.

PYRAMID EQUIVALENT: 2 ½ VEGETABLES, 3 OUNCES COOKED MEAT

Nutritional Analysis per Portion

calories 280 ▲ carbohydrate 23 grams ▲ protein 27 grams ▲ fat 9 grams
sodium 121 milligrams ▲ cholesterol 76 milligrams

▲▲

PENNE WITH BEANS AND GREENS

MAKES 4 PORTIONS

Red Swiss chard is an eye-catching green to use here. You can also use spinach, turnip greens, or even collards and kale (increase the cooking times for these two— or try frozen chopped collard greens, thawed). Teaming up pasta with beans and greens is a fiber-rich way to combine protein with some iron and beta carotene. Beans here count as a protein equivalent.

1 cup chicken or vegetable broth (see page 40)
1 tablespoon extra-virgin olive oil
2 large garlic cloves, minced
4 cups greens, cut into 1-inch strips, with about 1 inch of the stems included
2 cups cooked cannellini beans or 1 can (15 ounces), rinsed and drained
½ cup chopped red bell pepper
¾ teaspoon dried thyme, crumbled
¼ teaspoon crushed red pepper flakes, or to taste
8 ounces penne, cooked al dente
2 tablespoons grated Parmesan cheese

156

In a large, nonstick skillet heat the broth and oil over medium heat; add the garlic and cook for 1 minute. Stir in the remaining ingredients, except the pasta and cheese. Cover and cook for 3 to 8 minutes, depending on the greens (spinach cooks more quickly; collards and kale take longer).

In a large warmed serving bowl toss the greens and pasta together; sprinkle with cheese and serve.

PYRAMID EQUIVALENT: 2 BREADS, ½ VEGETABLE,
1 OUNCE MEAT ALTERNATE

Nutritional Analysis per Portion

calories 392 ▲ carbohydrate 67 grams ▲ protein 18 grams ▲ fat 6 grams
sodium 111 milligrams ▲ cholesterol 2 milligrams

▲▲

NO-FAT/NO-SWEAT LASAGNA WITH SPINACH AND LENTILS

MAKES 6 PORTIONS

I discovered the technique of *not* cooking the noodles—just layering them in the baking dish—when I was writing my microwave cookbook, *Quick Harvest*. You can buy special no-boil noodles, which cook a bit faster, but any brand will do the deed. Now that there are so many good reduced-salt and low-fat sauces in the super-market, I'm very prone to using them in a pinch. This really is *the* dish to make in the microwave, because it's done in less than 20 minutes, but I've included the conventional timing anyway.

Quick-cooking red lentils also steam themselves done here; and though some of the nonfat cheeses can be flat-tasting, they work well here because of all the other ingredients around them to keep them moist. You'll never miss the fat.

1 15-ounce container nonfat ricotta cheese
1 10-ounce package frozen chopped spinach, thawed and squeezed of excess water
½ cup frozen egg substitute, thawed
⅓ cup grated Parmesan cheese (see page 41)
¼ cup chopped fresh parsley
¼ teaspoon EACH ground nutmeg and crushed red pepper flakes
3½ cups Quick Tomato Sauce (page 128)
9 lasagna noodles, uncooked
¼ cup red lentils, uncooked
1½ cups shredded nonfat mozzarella cheese (6 ounces)

In a large bowl combine the ricotta cheese, spinach, egg substitute, 2 tablespoons of the Parmesan cheese, parsley, nutmeg, and pepper. Mix well until thoroughly blended.

Pour 1 cup of sauce into an 11 × 7 × 2-inch microwavable (glass) baking dish. Spread sauce evenly to cover the bottom of dish. Arrange 3 noodles in a single layer on top of the sauce. Spoon one-third of the spinach and ricotta mixture over the noodles; spread to make an even layer.

Sprinkle 2 tablespoons of the lentils over the top, and ½ cup of the mozzarella cheese, and the remaining Parmesan. Pour 1½ cups of the tomato sauce over cheeses. Arrange another layer of noodles on top. Repeat the layering, using the remaining ingredients (note that the top layer is spinach and ricotta mixture and mozzarella cheese only). Cover tightly with vented plastic wrap. Microwave on MEDIUM-HIGH for 18 to 20 minutes, or until noodles are just tender when pierced with the tip of a sharp knife and sauce is bubbly. Rotate twice during cooking. Let stand, covered, for 15 minutes.

Conventional Preparation:

Preheat oven to 350° F. Assemble lasagna as directed above. Cover tightly with aluminum foil. Bake for 1 hour; remove aluminum foil and bake 10 minutes longer. Let stand 10 minutes before cutting.

PYRAMID EQUIVALENT: 1 ½ BREADS, 1 ½ VEGETABLES,
1 ¼ MILK, ¼ OUNCE MEAT ALTERNATE

Nutritional Analysis per Portion

calories 285 ▲ carbohydrate 34 grams ▲ protein 30 grams ▲ fat 2 grams
sodium 509 milligrams ▲ cholesterol 8 milligrams

▲▲

SAFFRON-SCENTED RISOTTO WITH PORTOBELLO MUSHROOMS

MAKES 4 PORTIONS

"One of my happiest discoveries is that the pressure cooker can produce a wonderfully chewy risotto in about 5 minutes with hardly a stir," writes Lorna J. Sass in her book *Recipes from an Ecological Kitchen*. "Classic risottos normally take about 30 minutes of continual stirring," she also notes. Since I tried the pressure-cooker method, I have never stirred a risotto again.

Use a starchy short-grain rice like Arborio, which can be found in gourmet stores and many supermarkets. I like to use the wild Portobello mushroom in this recipe for its strong, assertive flavor. (To me, these mushrooms taste like juicy, tender meat.) You may certainly use the domestic ones if you prefer. If you're using canned broth—and are not able to find a low-sodium one—dilute it by half with water so the risotto isn't too salty.

1 tablespoon extra-virgin olive oil
1 cup thinly sliced leeks (white and green parts), thoroughly rinsed
2 cups Portobello mushrooms, cut into bite-size pieces
1 1/2 cups Arborio rice
4 to 5 cups vegetable or chicken broth (see page 40)*
1/4 cup chopped fresh Italian (flat-leaf) parsley
1/4 teaspoon saffron threads
1/2 teaspoon salt
1/4 cup grated Parmesan cheese
Freshly ground black pepper

In a 6-quart pressure cooker heat the oil over medium heat; stir in the leeks and cook for 1 minute. Stir in the mushrooms and cook 1 minute longer. Add the rice, stirring thoroughly to coat with the oil. Stir in 4 cups of the broth and the remaining ingredients, except the cheese and pepper. Lock the lid in place and bring to high pressure over high heat. Lower the heat just enough to maintain high pressure; cook 5 minutes longer. Reduce pressure immediately and remove the lid, making sure to tilt it away from you to allow excess steam to escape.

The risotto may be soupy (though it will continue to absorb liquid; if necessary, add a bit more broth). Stir in the cheese and ladle into shallow soup bowls. Sprinkle with freshly ground black pepper.

Stovetop Preparation:

In a large heavy skillet heat oil and follow directions up to addition of broth. Stir in 1/2 cup of the broth, and stir constantly until almost absorbed. Add remaining broth, 1/2 cup at a time, stirring constantly, until rice is al dente and mixture is soupy. Stir in cheese and serve as directed above.

* Use more broth if you prefer a loose, soupy risotto.

PYRAMID EQUIVALENT: 2 BREADS, 3/4 VEGETABLE

Nutritional Analysis per Portion

calories 373 ▲ carbohydrate 67 grams ▲ protein 8 grams ▲ fat 8 grams
sodium 381 milligrams ▲ cholesterol 4 milligrams

BLUSHING PINK RISOTTO WITH BAROLO WINE

MAKES 4 PORTIONS

The best risotto with Barolo I ever tasted was at Palio restaurant in New York City. This recipe was inspired by that Barolo Risotto and by Lorna Sass's eye-arresting crimson risotto. I added one of my favorite combinations for pasta sauce, beets, and red wine.

I sometimes stir in some small uncooked shrimp or bay scallops just as the risotto is finishing. If you're using a pressure cooker, make sure you retain the oil in this recipe to prevent clogging the pressure (vent) valve.

    1 tablespoon canola oil
    1 cup chopped onion
    2 large garlic cloves, minced
    1 1/2 cups Arborio rice
    1/2 cup grated beet (uncooked)
    3 to 4 cups vegetable or chicken broth (see page 40)*
    1 cup dry red wine, such as Barolo
    1/2 teaspoon salt
    1/4 cup grated Parmesan cheese
    1/4 cup chopped basil, plus some shredded leaves for garnish

In a 6-quart pressure cooker heat the oil over medium heat; stir in the onion and garlic, and cook for 1 minute. Pour in the rice, stirring thoroughly to coat with the oil. Add beet, 3 cups of the broth, and the remaining ingredients, except the cheese and basil. Lock the lid in place and bring to high pressure over high heat. Lower the heat just enough to maintain high pressure; cook 5 minutes longer. Reduce pressure immediately and remove the lid, making sure to tilt the cooker away from you to allow excess steam to escape.

* Use more broth if you prefer a loose, soupy risotto.

The risotto may be quite soupy (though it will continue to absorb liquid; if necessary, add a bit more broth). Stir in the cheese and basil; ladle into shallow soup bowls. Garnish with basil leaves if desired.

Stovetop Preparation:

In a large heavy skillet heat oil and follow directions up to addition of broth. Stir in ½ cup of the broth and stir constantly until almost absorbed. Add the wine, and the remaining broth, ½ cup at a time, stirring constantly, until rice is al dente and mixture is soupy. Stir in cheese and serve as directed above.

PYRAMID EQUIVALENT: 2 BREADS, ½ VEGETABLE

Nutritional Analysis per Portion

calories 416 ▲ carbohydrate 68 grams ▲ protein 8 grams ▲ fat 7 grams
sodium 390 milligrams ▲ cholesterol 4 milligrams

▲▲

BLACK BEAN CHILI WITH RED PEPPERS AND CORN

MAKES 8 PORTIONS

There's no missing the meat in this chili, once you learn the trick I discovered a few years ago: unsweetened cocoa powder lends a rich, "meaty" flavor to chilies and stews. For the really daring who go for incendiary dishes, try adding a whole dry habañero chili that Frieda's produce company in California is sending into many supermarkets. It takes just one or two to give you a five-alarm version. Stewed tomatoes are not essential here, but I find them a tad less bitter than canned tomatoes, and they make a nice addition to chili. A generous splash of balsamic vinegar or red wine just before serving does it justice, too. The beans in this recipe are counted as protein equivalents; they could also be counted as vegetables.

1 tablespoon plus 1 teaspoon extra-virgin olive oil
2 cups EACH chopped onion and red bell pepper
3 tablespoons mild chili powder
1 teaspoon EACH ground cumin and cuminseed
2 cups vegetable stock or water (see page 40)
2 14½-ounce cans no-salt-added stewed tomatoes
8 cups cooked black beans or 4 15-ounce cans, rinsed and drained
2 tablespoons unsweetened cocoa powder
½ teaspoon ground red pepper, or to taste
2 cups fresh corn kernels cut from the cob or frozen kernels
Yogurt Cream, for garnish, optional (page 65)
Chopped fresh cilantro, for garnish

In a large saucepan heat the oil over medium heat. Add the onions, and cook for 3 minutes; stir in the red pepper, chili powder, cumin, and cuminseed, and cook 3 minutes longer. Stir in the remaining ingredients, except the corn, Yogurt Cream, and cilantro, and bring just to a boil. Reduce heat, and simmer, uncovered, for 25 minutes. Stir in corn, and cook 5 minutes longer.

Ladle into soup bowls, and garnish with a dollop of Yogurt Cream, if desired, and chopped cilantro.

PYRAMID EQUIVALENT: 2 VEGETABLES, 2 OUNCES MEAT ALTERNATE

Nutritional Analysis per Portion

calories 349 ▲ carbohydrate 63 grams ▲ protein 19 grams ▲ fat 5 grams
sodium 58 milligrams ▲ cholesterol 0 milligrams

▲▲▲

VEGETARIAN STIR-FRY HUNAN-STYLE

MAKES 4 PORTIONS

If you haven't tried tofu, this combination of ginger and vegetables can be a good way to start. The Chinese province of Hunan is noted for its spicy specialties, and you can make this dish as hot or as mild as your palate dictates by merely adding some dried hot chili peppers for more heat, or substituting peanut oil for the chili oil for a tamer version. This recipe is especially easy because most of the vegetables are ready to use. Some hot cooked rice is the finishing touch.

2 teaspoons chili oil
2 cups 1-inch red bell pepper pieces
1 tablespoon minced fresh gingerroot
1 6-ounce package frozen pea pods, thawed (about 2 cups)
1 15-ounce can baby corn, drained (about 1¾ cups)
1 15-ounce can straw mushrooms, drained (about 1¼ cups)
⅓ cup vegetable broth (see page 40)
12 ounces firm tofu, cut into 1-inch cubes

In a large skillet or wok heat oil over medium-high heat for about 30 seconds. Add the red pepper and ginger; stir-fry for 2 minutes. Add the remaining ingredients except the broth and tofu; cook and toss for 2 minutes. Stir in the broth and tofu; cover and cook 3 minutes longer.

PYRAMID EQUIVALENT: 3 VEGETABLES, 1 OUNCE MEAT ALTERNATE

Nutritional Analysis per Portion

calories 285 ▲ carbohydrate 35 grams ▲ protein 19 grams ▲ fat 11 grams
sodium 511 milligrams ▲ cholesterol 0 milligrams

164

▲▲

VEGETABLE LO MEIN

MAKES 4 PORTIONS

Any combination of your favorite vegetables will do the trick here. If you want to boost the protein, you can also toss in some tofu, raw scallops, or thin strips of beef or pork when cooking the garlic. Try to get genuine lo mein noodles, which are not too hard to find in ethnic markets or in many supermarkets. They really add a wonderful note. If you like your noodles spicy, try using chili oil instead of the sesame or peanut oil listed below.

    8 ounces dried Chinese lo mein noodles or thin spaghetti
    2 teaspoons sesame or peanut oil
    3–4 large garlic cloves, minced
    6 medium asparagus spears, cut into 1-inch pieces
    1 cup thinly sliced onion
    2 cups chopped bok choy (use green leafy part with about 1 inch of the
        white part)
    1 cup EACH sliced mushrooms and shredded carrots
    2 tablespoons EACH reduced-sodium soy sauce and dry sherry

Cook noodles according to package directions; drain well. Cover with a double layer of damp paper towels; set aside.

In a large skillet or wok heat the oil over medium-high heat. Add the garlic and asparagus and stir-fry for 2 minutes; stir in the remaining vegetables and cook 2 to 3 minutes longer (add a few tablespoons water if mixture is too dry). Add the remaining ingredients and the reserved noodles; toss well to combine. Cook for a few minutes longer, until the noodles are heated through.

PYRAMID EQUIVALENT: 2 BREADS, 1 ½ VEGETABLES

Nutritional Analysis per Portion

calories 293 ▲ carbohydrate 54 grams ▲ protein 10 grams ▲ fat 3 grams
sodium 340 milligrams ▲ cholesterol 0 milligrams

▲▲

PAD THAI

MAKES 4 PORTIONS

Rice noodles are the foundation of this ubiquitous and spicy Thai dish. There are as many variations of pad thai as there are chefs. Some include strips of chicken, tofu, or dried and/or fresh shrimp. This version is strictly vegetarian, but any of the items above can add some protein, and other vegetables like asparagus, green beans, or mushrooms can be used. If you don't have any chili oil on hand, try some sesame or peanut oil and a generous pinch of ground red (cayenne) pepper instead.

8 ounces 1/4-inch-wide dried rice noodles
1/3 cup vegetable or chicken broth (see page 40)
5 teaspoons fish sauce (nam pla)*
1 teaspoon sugar
1 tablespoon fresh lime juice
3/4 teaspoon paprika
2 teaspoons chili oil
2 cups bean sprouts
4 scallions (green onions), cut into 2-inch shreds
1/4 cup EACH chopped fresh cilantro and basil
Cilantro leaves for garnish, optional

In a large saucepan bring 2 quarts water to a boil. Stir in noodles and cook for 30 seconds. Turn off heat and let noodles stand for 5 minutes, or until still firm to the bite. Drain.

In a measuring cup stir together the broth, fish sauce, sugar, lime juice, and paprika.

In a large nonstick skillet heat oil over medium heat. Stir in the broth mixture and cook for 1 minute. Add the remaining ingredients and the cooked noodles. Stir frequently and cook 1 minute longer, or until the noodles are heated through. Garnish with cilantro leaves, if desired.

* Available at Asian markets or in the ethnic foods section in some supermarkets.

PYRAMID EQUIVALENT: 1½ BREADS, 1¼ VEGETABLES

Nutritional Analysis per Portion

calories 267 ▲ carbohydrate 57 grams ▲ protein 3 grams ▲ fat 3 grams
sodium 13 milligrams ▲ cholesterol 0 milligrams

▲▲▲

CAJUN LENTIL CAKES

MAKES 4 PORTIONS

These spicy vegetable cakes are a nice way to get more lentils and fiber into your menus. Leave the purée somewhat chunky and use the Creamy Tarragon Dressing (page 127), for a nice accompaniment. If time doesn't permit, a good bottled salsa (like the Guiltless Gourmet brand) makes a colorful and zesty topping.

2 cups Lentil Purée (page 178)
¼ cup plus 1 tablespoon dried unseasoned breadcrumbs
¼ cup EACH chopped red onion and red bell pepper
2 tablespoons EACH reduced-calorie mayonnaise and fresh lime juice
1 teaspoon Dijon mustard
¼ teaspoon Tabasco sauce
2 tablespoons snipped fresh chives or 1½ teaspoons dried chives

In a large bowl combine all the ingredients until blended; do not overmix. Cover and refrigerate for 15 minutes. Shape mixture into 8 cakes, each about ¾ inch thick.

Spray a large nonstick skillet with nonstick cooking spray. Heat pan over medium heat. Cook cakes in two batches for about 3 minutes on each side. Wipe and re-spray skillet in between batches.

PYRAMID EQUIVALENTS: ½ BREAD, 2 OUNCES MEAT ALTERNATE

Nutritional Analysis per Portion

calories 225 ▲ carbohydrate 36 grams ▲ protein 15 grams ▲ fat 3 grams
sodium 159 milligrams ▲ cholesterol 2 milligrams

▲▲

DESSERTS

PRUNE PURÉE

APRICOT PURÉE

LENTIL PURÉE

LOW-FAT FUDGY BROWNIES

APRICOT TORTE

LEMON POPPY BUNDT CAKE

MIXED BERRY TART

DEEP DELICIOUS COCOA SQUARES

ANGEL FOOD CAKE

CHOCOLATE ANGEL FOOD CAKE

PLUM GOOD BREAD PUDDING

GLAZED APPLES AND RAISINS

▲▲

"For those of us who love sweets too much for our own good, the discovery of no-fat baking ranks right up there with the discovery of penicillin," said food and health writer Marian Burros, in one of her *New York Times* "Eating Well" columns.

Luckily we are in an age when very delicious low-fat desserts are a dream that came true. Even more fortunate, as home bakers we can use all-natural ingredients and still have our cake and eat it too. And after all, why shouldn't we?

Whenever people are trying to cut back, cut down, or modify their eating, desserts are usually the first items to go. What a mistake. Desserts are truly fun; they're something we all look forward to, and they add to the festivity of any occasion. However, they're usually loaded with fat and sugar, and it's the fat that can really be devastating. Often butter, eggs, and cream are the ingredients that contain fat and cholesterol. Most of their fat is saturated and that tends to raise blood cholesterol.

But when we allow the concept of moderation to be part of our plans, and when we take a look at the Pyramid, we find there are no No's. That means the prudent use of ingredients like eggs and butter is absolutely permissible. And some common sense must also prevail. For instance, if you're preparing a cake or tart that contains one or two eggs and a few tablespoons of butter or oil to serve eight or ten people, the actual amount of fat per person may come out to be only one or two grams of fat. The taste and texture of the dessert will be far superior to one that is completely fat-free. This is the pleasure concept at work. Sometimes small amounts of so-called "forbidden" foods create a much better dish and enhance our enjoyment immensely.

Some folks will insist on fat-free food whenever possible. Remember that there are trade-offs on texture and sometimes on flavor when fat is absent in home-baked goods. Commercial items purchased at the supermarket contain special emulsifiers, gums, and ingredients not available to home bakers. This makes some commercial cakes or cookies virtually impossible to reproduce at home. That's why results are often disappointing when you try to make completely fat-free desserts in your kitchen. The very nature and chemical composition of fat is very distinctive: fat carries flavor; it "shortens" the dough and acts as a tenderizer; and it lends color and crispness to the final result.

My own choice is to keep some of the fat and also keep the pleasure. I even believe an occasional splurge for a full-fat ice cream or rich pastry is worth it when you have an overwhelming longing for it. By allowing yourself a treat on occasion, you avoid setting yourself up for the binges that may result from too much deprivation.

The recipes here include a smidgen of fat and, as you'll see, other ingredients like fruit purées and nonfat yogurt. The results are impressive. If you are determined to get all the fat out, so be it.

Granulated or confectioners' sugar and fruit purées are the primary sweeteners used. I think you'll find the desserts are pleasantly sweet, but not cloyingly so; nor are they dull and flat. In recipes where a cup of sugar is called for, look at the number of servings. It will likely serve ten—or more—and that's about 1½ table-spoons of sugar per serving.

I encourage everyone to have more fruit—fresh, canned in natural juices, and frozen—for dessert. But when you're inclined to bake or have a special request, these recipes will deliver flavor without much fat.

Egg whites lighten both the Angel Food Cake and the Chocolate Angel Food Cake—desserts without any fat at all. The Lemon Poppy Bundt Cake is one of my favorites. It's made with just 3 tablespoons of oil, applesauce, and egg whites, yet it tastes as rich as one that uses several whole eggs and a quarter pound of butter. Chocolate lovers will relish the Low-Fat Fudgy Brownies made with prune purée, cocoa powder, and vegetable oil. No one will miss the butter and eggs, nor will they detect the presence of prunes.

Glazed Apples and Raisins will delight all the fruit lovers at your house. You can make this simple dessert on top of the stove or in the microwave in less than fifteen minutes. For those who are fans of bread pudding, the Plum Good Bread Pudding is the one to make. No whole eggs or cream here either. Apple juice, unsweetened applesauce, and egg whites provide for a pudding of stellar quality.

There are no forbidden foods in the Pyramid guidelines, so there's no reason to forgo desserts. You will always want to keep a judicious eye on the amount of fat they contain, then balance it with the rest of what you eat. You also need to keep in mind the sugar content. As trim as the desserts are here, they are made with sugar. So keep a watchful eye in order to avoid excess.

TIPS FOR BETTER BAKING

▲ Preheat oven *before* mixing cake or muffins. Baking soda or baking powder, two ingredients that make baked products rise, begin to work as soon as they are mixed with the liquid ingredients. It is essential to pop the batters into a preheated oven to allow the heat to do the rest of the job.

▲ Use an oven thermometer. In many home ovens the number on the outside dial may have nothing at all to do with the actual temperature inside the oven. Baking in an oven that is too cool or too hot will produce very disappointing results. To avoid this, hang the thermometer in the center of the shelf that is closest to where the pan will sit during baking. The shelf should be in the middle of the oven, unless indicated otherwise in the recipe. Get to know your oven too. It may be perfectly accurate at 350° F, but when you turn the dial to 425° F the thermometer may register 475° F. Temperature and timing are especially crucial in low-fat baking, where dry, tough products are what you'll end up with if they are overbaked.

▲ Measure carefully for the best results. Use the measuring cups and spoons that come in nested sets for measuring dry ingredients and use calibrated glass or plastic measuring cups for liquid ingredients. Use a fork or whisk to aerate the flour (it may have packed down in the canister); then scoop it into a measuring cup and sweep or level it off with the blunt edge of a knife. When the dry ingredients are measured into the bowl I find that whisking is an excellent way to combine ingredients and sifting is unnecessary (most flours today are presifted anyway). Cake flour, however, should be sifted *before* measuring for best results.

▲ Try using fruit juices or water in which you've cooked the fruit for all or part of the liquid in recipes. The low-fat and nonfat versions of buttermilk, yogurt, and sour cream also do a lot for improving flavor and texture.

▲ Reduce sweeteners and salt in the recipes if you must, but don't eliminate them altogether. Both bring out the full flavors of the ingredients and, in the case of yeast breads, sugar is essential in "feeding" the yeast so the dough will rise properly.

▲ For each whole egg, substitute two egg whites or an equivalent of frozen egg substitute (usually ¼ cup per egg, but check the label of the brand you're using).

▲ When using low-fat buttermilk, use baking soda rather than baking powder for leavening.

▲ Spray pans and muffin tins with nonstick cooking spray instead of coating with butter or oil. Wax paper and parchment paper can also be placed in the sprayed pan for cakes that have a long cooking time.

▲ Time recipes carefully. A kitchen timer with a loud buzzer is the best insurance against overcooking. Once something is overbaked there's no going back.

▲ Test for doneness by inserting a wooden toothpick or special cake tester in the center of the cake. When it comes out clean the cake is done (unless instructions suggest otherwise). Baking times given in recipes are not gospel. Every oven is different.

▲ Use wire racks for cooling. They protect table and counter tops when cakes are cooling in the pan for the first few minutes they're out of the oven, and they allow a free flow of air.

LOWERING OR ELIMINATING FAT—BETTER IN ANY EVENT

When you're converting your favorite recipe, enhance the results by trying these tricks.

▲ Use cake flour for all or part of the flour called for in the recipe. Substitute 1 cup plus 2 tablespoons *sifted* cake flour for each cup of all-purpose flour.

▲ Do not overmix low-fat or fat-free batters. Fat helps to tenderize and coat the strands of gluten (protein) in flour. When fat is absent strands can break, making the cake or muffin tough and rubbery.

▲ Use fruit purées and fat-free fruit butters (available in health food stores or in the jelly section of the supermarket) in equal amounts for fat. Recipes are provided for prune and apricot purée on the following pages; any of your other favorite dried fruits can be used.

▲ Use unsweetened applesauce, canned pumpkin (not pumpkin pie mix, which has spices added to it), and puréed fruit or vegetable baby food in jars as other replacements for fat.

▲ Try fresh fruits as well as dried ones. Soft fruits like banana, mango, and papaya work quite well in the same one-to-one proportions for fat.

▲ Use European-style cocoa in recipes that call for unsweetened cocoa powder. It is made with alkali, which brings up the chocolate flavor and enriches the color.

DON'T STOP WITH FRUITS

Try using puréed or vegetable baby foods for savory baked goods like corn bread or carrot muffins.

Pumpkin and cooked dried lentils or split peas also make excellent replacements in baking recipes. I prefer canned pumpkin rather than fresh pumpkin. It is more consistent, easier to handle, and already has the ideal amount of water extracted from it to give you dependable results every time. Substitute vegetable purées for fat in the same one-to-one ratio as fruit purées.

Lentils will add fiber, protein, and extra moistness to your baked goods. Keep lentil purée covered and refrigerated; once it is made, it should last about a week. It also freezes very well if you'd like to keep it longer. Put it in an airtight plastic container when you do.

▲ One pound of split peas make about 6 cups of purée.

▲ One pound of lentils makes about 7 cups of purée.

FRUIT PURÉES

One day, out of the blue, what looked like a brownie, along with a box of prunes, some press materials, and a recipe brochure arrived from the California Prune Board. I glanced at the press release that touted the merits of the brownie I was about to bite into and became a bit dubious. Prunes in a brownie? But it was quite good. The test kitchens of the California Prune Board had come up with a satisfactory *and* easy recipe that allowed folks like you and me to make moist and delicious low-fat brownies at home. The secret was prune purée.

The simple method is to purée dried pitted prunes and water in a food processor or blender until smooth and use this concoction to replace all of the fat in a direct one-to-one substitution in baked goods. Prune butter, which is conveniently available in the jam and jelly section, or the baking section of most supermarkets, and in health food stores, is a handy alternative. Using prune purée in baked goods may cut fat by as much as 75 to 90 percent, calories by 20 to 30 percent, and cholesterol to zero. Whatever traces of fat that might remain come from other ingredients like unsweetened chocolate (or oil blended with cocoa powder) or chopped nuts.

The magic is that the taste of prunes is virtually imperceptible after they are mixed and cooked with other ingredients. What's even better is that the prunes add fiber, iron, vitamin A, and potassium. It took no time at all for the media to catch on and promote the idea. Newspaper and magazine test kitchens everywhere started developing recipes that even novice bakers could use at home to make delicious cookies, cakes, and muffins. At last it looks like the door to more palatable low-fat and fat-free baking has swung open.

In the few years since that first prune brownie arrived at my door, I have followed the developments closely and have worked extensively with dried fruit purées, applesauce, baby-food fruits, lentil purée, and nonfat yogurt as substitutes for fat. I have had very good results using just one substitute like applesauce, and equally good results using a combination—like applesauce and nonfat yogurt—in the same recipe. You might also consider using other dried fruit purées such as fig, peach, or nectarine. By all means, be adventurous. I'm certain there are all sorts of pleasing results you can achieve with a little experimenting.

▲▲▲

PRUNE PURÉE

MAKES 1 CUP

This may become one of the classic fat replacements of all times. It's one I'm sure you'll want to use in a number of ways. It works well in cakes, muffins, quick breads, and of course, in Low-Fat Fudgy Brownies (page 179).

1 1/3 cups (8 ounces) dried pitted prunes
6 tablespoons water

In a food processor or blender combine the prunes and water until prunes are finely chopped and the mixture has the consistency of a purée.

Store in an airtight container in the refrigerator for up to one month.

PYRAMID EQUIVALENT (PER 1/4 CUP): 1 FRUIT

Nutritional Analysis per 1/4 Cup

calories 136 ▲ carbohydrate 36 grams ▲ protein 2 grams ▲ fat 0 grams
sodium 2 milligrams ▲ cholesterol 0 milligrams

▲▲▲

APRICOT PURÉE

MAKES 1 CUP

This makes a wonderful ingredient for the Cinnamon-scented Apricot Bread (page 54) as a substitution for all or part of the applesauce. I add a touch of vanilla to this purée to round out the flavor.

1 1/3 cups dried apricots (about 8 ounces)
5 tablespoons water
1/2 teaspoon vanilla

In a food processor or blender combine the apricots, water, and vanilla until apricots are finely chopped and the mixture has the consistency of a purée.

Store in an airtight container in the refrigerator for up to one month.

▲▲

· LENTIL PURÉE

MAKES ABOUT 2 CUPS

You can use this recipe in myriad ways. I sometimes add thyme, marjoram, or nutmeg to make it a dip for hors d'oeuvres or use a pastry bag and pipe it around the edge of a serving platter as a garnish. I use it to add fiber and flavor to muffins and quick breads when I'm reducing fat. This purée freezes well. You can also substitute dried split peas for the lentils.

1 cup dried lentils, rinsed and drained
2½ cups water

In a medium saucepan combine lentils and water. Cover, and bring to a boil. Reduce heat, and simmer for 40 to 45 minutes, or until lentils are quite soft, stirring occasionally.

Cool slightly; do not drain. In a food processor or blender (you can also use a food mill or sieve), purée the lentils until they are the consistency of canned pumpkin. Add additional water, if necessary.

PYRAMID EQUIVALENT (PER ½ CUP):
1 VEGETABLE, 1 OUNCE MEAT ALTERNATE

· Nutritional Analysis per ½ Cup

calories 162 ▲ carbohydrate 27 grams ▲ protein 13 grams ▲ fat 0 grams
sodium 5 milligrams ▲ cholesterol 0 milligrams

▲▲▲

LOW-FAT FUDGY BROWNIES

MAKES 3 DOZEN BROWNIES

Here they are—the brownies from California that made baking history. You'll rave about these bite-size treats that are made with prune purée instead of butter and whole eggs.

3/4 cup unsweetened cocoa powder
1/4 cup canola oil
1/2 cup Prune Purée (page 176) or prune butter
3 large egg whites, at room temperature
1 cup sugar
1/2 teaspoon salt
1 teaspoon vanilla
1/2 cup all-purpose flour
1/4 cup chopped walnuts, optional

Preheat oven to 350° F. Spray an 8-inch square baking pan with nonstick cooking spray; set aside.

In a medium bowl, using an electric mixer on low speed, combine all the ingredients except the flour and walnuts (if using); beat to blend. Stir in the flour. Scrape the batter into the pan; sprinkle with nuts, if using.

Bake for 30 minutes, or until the top edges about 2 inches from the center spring back when gently touched with the tip of the finger. Cool brownies in pan, on a wire rack. Cut into 36 squares.

Nutritional Analysis per Brownie (without nuts)

calories 55 ▲ carbohydrate 10 grams ▲ protein 1 gram ▲ fat 2 grams
sodium 35 milligrams ▲ cholesterol 0 milligrams

▲▲▲

APRICOT TORTE

MAKES 8 PORTIONS

Though it's called an apricot torte, this recipe can be made with almost any fruit you like, depending on what's in season. Peaches and apples are good substitutes for the apricots, as are small prune plums available in early fall. This dessert is good accompanied by low-fat vanilla yogurt, fruit-flavored frozen yogurt, or lemon sherbet.

3/4 cup Apricot Purée (page 177), or one 6-ounce jar baby-food apricots
1 egg
1/2 cup plus 1 teaspoon sugar
1 cup all-purpose flour
1 teaspoon grated lemon peel (yellow part only), optional
3/4 teaspoon baking powder
1/4 teaspoon ground cardamom
2 cups small, ripe apricots, halved and pitted (about 1 pound)

Preheat oven to 350° F.

Spray a 9-inch springform pan with nonstick cooking spray; set aside.

In a medium bowl, using an electric mixer on low speed, beat together the apricot purée, egg, and 1/2 cup of the sugar until blended. Beat in flour, lemon peel, baking powder, and cardamom. Pour batter into prepared pan; smooth to make an even layer. Place apricots together, skin side down, in concentric circles; sprinkle with remaining teaspoon of sugar.

Bake for 35 to 40 minutes, or until puffy and a tester inserted in center of dough comes out clean. Place pan on a wire rack to cool. Run the tip of a sharp knife around the edges of the pan; loosen and remove sides of the pan, and serve. Serve warm, or at room temperature.

PYRAMID EQUIVALENT: ½ BREAD, ¾ FRUIT (FOR APRICOT PURÉE)
OR ½ FRUIT (FOR BABY FOOD)

Nutritional Analysis per Portion

calories 194 ▲ carbohydrate 44 grams ▲ protein 4 grams ▲ fat 1 gram
sodium 57 milligrams ▲ cholesterol 27 milligrams

▲▲

LEMON POPPY BUNDT CAKE

MAKES 1 CAKE; 12 PORTIONS

Serve this moist, attractive cake with pride at any special occasion. It will rival any butter- and egg-laden cake you've ever made. Even the sugar has been reduced here, so there's less than 2 tablespoons per serving.

1½ cups EACH all-purpose flour and sifted cake flour
1½ cups sugar
2 teaspoons baking powder
1 teaspoon baking soda
¾ teaspoon salt
1½ cups unsweetened applesauce
3 tablespoons EACH vegetable oil and fresh lemon juice
1 tablespoon grated lemon peel (yellow part only)
4 egg whites, at room temperature
¼ cup poppy seeds

Preheat oven to 350° F. Spray a 10-cup bundt pan with nonstick cooking spray; set aside.

In a large bowl whisk together the flours, 1 cup of the sugar, baking powder, baking soda, and salt; set aside.

In a medium bowl whisk together the applesauce, oil, lemon juice, and lemon peel until blended.

In another medium bowl, using an electric mixer on high speed, beat the egg whites until foamy and almost double in volume. Slowly beat in the remaining ½ cup of sugar until whites form soft peaks.

Make a well in the center of the flour mixture. Pour in applesauce mixture, and stir until just combined. (Mixture will be quite thick.) Stir about ¼ of the egg whites into the batter; gently fold remaining egg whites into the batter and fold in poppy seeds. Pour batter into prepared pan; shake gently to distribute batter evenly.

Bake for 35 minutes, or until a tester inserted in center comes out clean. Cool in pan on a wire rack for 5 minutes; turn onto rack to finish cooling.

PYRAMID EQUIVALENT: 1 ¼ BREADS, ¼ FRUIT

Nutritional Analysis per Portion

calories 263 ▲ carbohydrate 51 grams ▲ protein 4 grams ▲ fat 5 grams
sodium 345 milligrams ▲ cholesterol 0 milligrams

▲▲▲

MIXED BERRY TART

MAKES 6 PORTIONS

Here's one of those recipes that deserves to keep the butter. The amount used is a bit more than a tablespoon per serving, and it's well worth it. There's no rich pastry cream here, just pure, fresh berries and a touch of red currant jelly painted on the crust to pull all the flavors together. Anyone can make this easy dessert, which comes from my friend Jane Cooper.

1 cup all-purpose flour
7 tablespoons sweet butter, softened
1/3 cup plus 2 tablespoons sugar
1 tablespoon white vinegar
2 cups blueberries
1 cup raspberries
1/4 teaspoon ground cinnamon
1 tablespoon red currant jelly, at room temperature

Preheat oven to 375° F.

In a medium bowl combine the flour, butter, 2 tablespoons of the sugar, and vinegar with your hands until the mixture holds together. Press into a round disk and place in the center of a 9-inch tart pan. Refrigerate for 5 minutes. Pat the dough with your fingertips until it evenly covers the bottom and sides of the pan. (While working, wet fingertips with cool water if the dough gets too sticky.)

Using the same bowl combine the remaining 1/3 cup sugar with 1 1/2 cups of the blueberries, 1/2 cup of the raspberries, and cinnamon. Brush the jelly over the bottom of the tart; pour berry mixture into the pan and shake to make an even layer.

Bake for 50 minutes, or until the berries are soft. Remove from oven, and place the remaining berries over the top. Gently press to make an even layer. Let the tart cool. Remove the rim of the pan and serve.

PYRAMID EQUIVALENT: 1 BREAD, 1/2 FRUIT

Nutritional Analysis per Portion

calories 299 ▲ carbohydrate 43 grams ▲ protein 3 grams ▲ fat 14 grams

sodium 6 milligrams ▲ cholesterol 36 milligrams

▲▲

DEEP DELICIOUS COCOA SQUARES

MAKES 16 PORTIONS

I used to make this cake with sour cream, three eggs, butter, and chocolate and then slather on a rich buttercream frosting to top it off. But evaporated skimmed milk, 2 eggs, applesauce, and cocoa powder make this slimmed-down version as tasty as ever. It's so good that icing really isn't necessary; a simple dusting with confectioners' sugar does quite nicely.

  2 cups all-purpose flour
  2 cups sugar
  ³/₄ cup unsweetened Dutch-process cocoa powder
  1 ¹/₂ teaspoons baking soda
  1 teaspoon baking powder
  ¹/₂ teaspoon salt
  1 cup unsweetened applesauce
  1 cup evaporated skimmed milk
  2 eggs
  Confectioners' sugar, optional

Preheat oven to 350° F. Spray a 12 × 9-inch baking pan with nonstick cooking spray; set aside.

In a large bowl whisk together the flour, sugar, cocoa powder, baking soda, baking powder, and salt; set aside.

In a medium bowl whisk together the applesauce, milk, and eggs. Make a well in the center of the flour mixture. Pour in applesauce mixture, and stir until just combined. Do not overmix. Pour batter into prepared pan. Bake for 40 to 45 minutes, or until a tester inserted in center comes out clean. Cool in pan.

Sprinkle lightly with confectioners' sugar, if desired, and cut into 16 squares.

▲▲▲

ANGEL FOOD CAKE

MAKES 1 CAKE; 12 PORTIONS

High, light, and fluffy are the characteristics of angel food cakes. Fat-free and cholesterol-free, they are as versatile as can be. Serve this one at any occasion plain, garnished with fresh fruit, or with Blueberry Sauce (page 130), which is sublime. Should there be any left over, it's yummy when lightly toasted.

It is important that eggs be carefully separated so not a trace of egg yolk remains—otherwise the whites just won't beat up well. Both beaters and bowl must also be absolutely free of any fat or grease to give the cake its best results.

Use two forks or a comblike metal cake divider (designed for angel food cakes) to gently pull the cake apart and serve it. I find that a serrated bread knife makes easy work of slicing too.

Angel food cake is a great make-ahead dessert as it stores well when tightly wrapped. It does not, however, freeze very well.

1¼ cups superfine sugar
1 cup plus 2 tablespoons sifted cake flour
12 large egg whites, at room temperature
1 teaspoon cream of tartar
½ teaspoon salt
2 teaspoons vanilla

Preheat oven to 375° F.

In a medium bowl whisk together ¾ cup of the sugar and the cake flour; set aside.

In a large bowl, using an electric mixer at medium speed, beat egg whites until thick and foamy. Increase speed to high; add cream of tartar, salt, and vanilla. Continue beating until soft peaks form. Gradually sprinkle the remaining ½ cup sugar over the top and continue beating on high speed, until peaks are glossy and stiff, but not dry and overbeaten.

Gently and quickly fold in flour mixture in three batches, using a rubber spatula, slotted spoon, or large balloon whisk. Pour into an *ungreased* 10-inch tube pan with removable sides; run a sharp knife through the batter to break any air pockets.

Bake for 30 to 35 minutes, or until a tester inserted in center comes out clean.

Hang the cake inverted on a wine bottle or funnel or invert on a wire rack and cool completely. Run a thin metal spatula or sharp knife around the sides and release from pan.

Nutritional Analysis per Portion

calories 133 ▲ carbohydrate 29 grams ▲ protein 4 grams ▲ fat 0 grams
sodium 146 milligrams ▲ cholesterol 0 milligrams

▲▲▲

CHOCOLATE ANGEL FOOD CAKE

MAKES 1 CAKE; 12 PORTIONS

Know that there will be requests for seconds on this luscious yet guilt-free chocolate cake. Cocoa powder contains no fat, and using a Dutch-process, or European-style, cocoa lends a smoother flavor and richer color to the cake. I believe that chocolate recipes should be prepared the night before you plan to serve them so that all the flavors soften.

1 1/3 cups superfine sugar

1 cup sifted cake flour

1/3 cup unsweetened cocoa powder

14 large egg whites, at room temperature

1 1/2 teaspoons cream of tartar

1/4 teaspoon salt

2 teaspoons Triple Sec, optional

1 1/2 teaspoons vanilla

Preheat oven to 350° F.

In a medium bowl whisk together 2/3 cup of the sugar, flour, and cocoa powder.

In a large bowl, using an electric mixer at medium speed, beat egg whites until thick and foamy. Increase speed to high; add cream of tartar, salt, Triple Sec (if using), and vanilla. Continue beating until soft peaks form. Gradually sprinkle the remaining 2/3 cup sugar over the top and continue beating on high speed, until peaks are glossy and stiff, but not dry and overbeaten.

Gently and quickly fold in flour mixture in three batches using a rubber spatula, slotted spoon, or large balloon whisk. Pour into an *ungreased* 10-inch tube pan with removable sides; run a sharp knife through the batter to break any air pockets.

Bake for 40 minutes, or until a tester inserted in center comes out clean.

Hang the cake inverted on a wine bottle or funnel; or invert on a wire rack and cool completely. Run a thin metal spatula or sharp knife around the sides and release from pan.

Nutritional Analysis per Portion

calories 143 ▲ carbohydrate 30 grams ▲ protein 5 grams ▲ fat 0 grams

sodium 110 milligrams ▲ cholesterol 0 milligrams

▲▲

PLUM GOOD BREAD PUDDING

MAKES 6 PORTIONS

I'm a real fan of the small, soft purple prune plums that appear early in September. You needn't limit this yummy no-fat dessert to prune plums only. Use an equal amount of your favorite fruit, and by all means vary the type of juice or nectar as well.

1 1/2 cups unsweetened applesauce
3/4 cup apple juice
1 cup evaporated skimmed milk
4 egg whites
1/3 cup packed light brown sugar
1 teaspoon ground cinnamon
1/2 teaspoon ground cardamom
9 ounces stale bread (about 7 cups), cut or torn into 1-inch pieces
2 1/2 cups prune plums, halved and pitted (about 3/4 pound)

Preheat oven to 350° F.

In a 3-quart oval casserole gently whisk together applesauce, apple juice, milk, egg whites, sugar, cinnamon, and cardamom until sugar is dissolved and mixture is frothy. Stir in bread cubes and plums. Let stand for 20 minutes. Meanwhile, bring about 4 cups of water to a boil.

Place casserole in a large baking pan and pour boiling water in the pan until it comes about halfway up the sides of casserole. With a whisk or the back of a spoon, gently press down bread mixture. Bake for 40 minutes, or until a knife inserted in the center comes out clean. Let stand for 10 minutes before serving.

Microwave Preparation:

Cover casserole with vented plastic wrap and place in oven (a water bath is not needed). Microwave on HIGH for 3 minutes; reduce setting to MEDIUM and micro-wave for 15 minutes, or until it tests done.

Nutritional Analysis per Portion

calories 286 ▲ carbohydrate 59 grams ▲ protein 10 grams ▲ fat 2 grams
sodium 321 milligrams ▲ cholesterol 2 milligrams

▲▲▲

GLAZED APPLES AND RAISINS

MAKES 4 PORTIONS

Think of this as apple pie without the pastry. It's lovely served on its own, with frozen yogurt, or with Angel Food Cake (page 185). Best of all, it's ready in less than 15 minutes, and about half that when cooked in the microwave. Peel the apples if you like, but I prefer to leave the skins on and get the extra fiber. I also like to use several kinds of apples, like McIntosh, Golden Delicious, and Granny Smith, all at the same time.

2 teaspoons sweet butter
1 teaspoon canola oil
¾ teaspoon ground cinnamon
½ teaspoon ground ginger
¼ teaspoon ground cloves
3 large apples, cored and cut into ½-inch slices (about 1 ½ pounds)
¾ cup orange juice
¼ cup golden raisins

In a large nonstick skillet heat the butter and oil over medium heat; stir in the cinnamon, ginger, and cloves until blended. Stir in the apples, and cook, stirring constantly to coat the apples evenly with the spice mixture, for 2 minutes. Add the remaining ingredients. Reduce heat, cover partially, and simmer for about 10 minutes, or until the apples are tender. Remove from heat. Let cool slightly and serve warm, or at room temperature.

Microwave Preparation:

In a shallow 3-quart microwavable casserole combine the butter, oil, cinnamon, ginger, and cloves; microwave on HIGH, uncovered, for 1 minute. Stir in the remaining ingredients. Cover partially with lid or vented plastic wrap. Microwave on MEDIUM-HIGH for 6 minutes, or until apples are almost tender. Let stand for 2 minutes.

PYRAMID EQUIVALENT: 2 FRUITS

Nutritional Analysis per Portion

calories 170 ▲ carbohydrate 37 grams ▲ protein 1 gram ▲ fat 4 grams
sodium 2 milligrams ▲ cholesterol 5 milligrams

SUPERMARKETS GET SAVVY

There's no question that we are all eating out more. Statistics bear out the fact that an increasing portion of the food dollar is being spent outside the home. But there's little doubt that what we buy at the supermarket still influences most of what we eat each day. Food shopping, then, is an important part of eating within the framework of the Pyramid and the Dietary Guidelines. The Pyramid can help you plan menus and plan what you're going to buy before you go to the supermarket. Either make a shopping list or keep variety and moderation in mind. That way you'll select foods that provide the protein, vitamins, minerals, carbohydrates, and fiber you need for good health.

No one knows more about being a savvy supermarket shopper than Leni Reed. Ms. Reed is a registered dietitian and head of Leni Reed Associates, Inc./Supermarket Savvy in Reston, Virginia. For years she has been leading consumer tours in supermarkets, teaching people how to make more healthful food choices. She has trained countless numbers of home economists, nutritionists, and other professionals to lead these same tours in areas all across America. Her goal is to help people *know* what they are buying so that they can stick to weight or health plans they've established, and not get caught in the pitfalls of shrewd advertising and marketing ploys. She literally takes people through the aisles and examines food products along the way. People get firsthand instruction on how to read labels, how to judge fact from fiction, and how to save money. Leni and her associates publish a national newsletter six times a year to look at new products that are nationally distributed (see page 229). Simply Eggs, Bisquick Reduced Fat Variety Baking and Pancake Mix, and Mazola RightBlend oil are a few of the many products reviewed in one issue. Readers find out what's on the label, how it compares to a similar product (like how the Reduced Fat Bisquick mixes compare with the original), what sizes are available, and the suggested retail price. The "At a Glance" section includes clear and informative charts that give an overall look at a category of food, like frozen entrées. Several brands are listed with the nutrition information for each in a handy chart form.

Lots of other tips are included, and each issue has a section called "Worth Writing or Calling For" that refers readers to resources for more information they can get for free or at a nominal charge. Twice each year the "Supermarket Savvy Brand Name Shopping List" is updated. This is a comprehensive list of the healthiest foods, from cereals to crackers, from salad dressings to cheeses—by brand names. It lists foods that are low in fat, saturated fat, cholesterol, sodium, and sugar, and high in fiber. Though the newsletter was originally marketed for health professionals, consumers may contact the company for more information about it and the brand-name list.

WHAT'S GOING ON IN SUPERMARKETS

It's encouraging to see how many of the supermarkets all around the country responded to the release of the Food Guide Pyramid. Many of them jumped right on the bandwagon in getting the word out to their customers. Signs, posters, and brochures were developed to get their shoppers better acquainted with the Pyramid and to help them shop with a sharper eye toward health. Here's what some of the stores are doing.

Safeway Inc. has used the Food Pyramid in their nutrition newsletter and tailored it to the needs of children. Their future plans include production of a Food Guide Pyramid pamphlet and possible use of the Pyramid with in-store point-of-sale programs in the bakery, produce, and meat departments. Safeway Inc. operates nine hundred supermarkets in seventeen states. Their efforts in this area are by no means new. In response to consumer interest in health and nutrition information they implemented a nutrition awareness program in 1982 that included a full-color food-and-nutrition newsletter published six times a year and monthly nutrition pamphlets (see page 229). Safeway's nutrition programs strive to increase consumer awareness of the relationships among food, diet, and health, based on the Dietary Guidelines for Americans. It's no surprise then that they would concur with the Food Guide Pyramid recommendations.

On the East Coast **Stop & Shop** stores are committed to providing relevant nutritional information to customers. After an extensive study, 90 percent of the shoppers at Stop & Shop said that nutrition information was important to them. They also said that eating nutritious foods is the primary key to staying healthy; and 81 percent indicated they were extremely or very concerned about fat. The "Leaner Choice Guide to Low Fat Shopping" program was developed and designed to provide shelf labeling for products that meet government-proposed definitions of "fat-free," "low in fat," and "reduced fat." Stop & Shop also has specific food guides for each department in the store. All of the 119 stores are participating in a program that mirrors the instruction of the Dietary Guidelines and the Food Pyramid.

Rochester, New York–based **Wegmans** food markets have put the Food Pyramid on some of their private-label food packages. Starting in the Bread, Cereal, Rice, and Pasta Group, Wegmans began a program called "Food You Feel Good About." Packages in the bakery department carry instructions on how to store and serve the Wegmans baked breads. In addition each bag has a picture of the Pyramid and provides examples of what a serving from the bread group might be. Wegmans included a graphic of the Pyramid in their advertising, and colorful paper danglers hang in the store to highlight the Pyramid and the "Food You Feel Good About" items.

The 77 **Price Chopper** stores, which are based in Schenectady, New York, developed the "Eat Wise, Health Wise" booklet for their shoppers. This handy leaflet shows the Pyramid and includes information on how to read food labels, with an emphasis on choosing foods that are low in fat, cholesterol, and sodium and high in fiber. It also includes low-fat cooking tips. Along with Healthy Choice, Nabisco, and other food companies, Price Chopper conducted in-store cholesterol screenings free of charge. The brochure was distributed and registered dietitians were available for consultation.

Giant Foods, in the Washington, D.C., area, targeted a Pyramid education program to children and parents through their "Healthy Start . . . Food to Grow On" campaign. The program is aimed at families with young kids ages two to six. All 155 stores distributed a newsletter explaining the Pyramid to parents. Parents were reminded that a two- to four-year-old will not eat the portion sizes of the Pyramid and that the key is to cover all groups. Giant's newsletter suggested a handy rule of thumb as one tablespoon of each food for each year of age, except for milk; children should get the equivalent of two 8-ounce glasses. The suggestion offered for foods like bread and meat, which are not measured in tablespoons, is to try half portions, such as a half to three-quarters of a slice of bread, 1 to 2 ounces of meat, etc. The newsletter also invited children to make their own Food Pyramid Poster. The *Eater's Almanac*, a publication distributed to adult shoppers, devoted an entire issue to the Food Guide Pyramid.

Many of the markets are teaming the Pyramid with their 5 a Day promotions. **Pratt Foods**, in Oklahoma City, used the Food Pyramid as a nutrition marketing tool for produce. J. B. Pratt, the president of the company, developed a large three-dimensional Food Guide Pyramid model for display in his produce departments.

Look around in your area. Retailers everywhere are more and more committed to providing information, in-store demos, classes, home economists, and even registered dietitians to help shoppers select foods to encourage a healthful diet.

A STROLL THROUGH THE AISLES—GET SOME SAVVY OF YOUR OWN

Smart shoppers know that there are lots of good, wholesome foods to choose from in the supermarket. Many frozen, packaged, and canned "convenience" items fit in very well with the guidelines of the Food Pyramid. It can still be something of a challenge to find them though, since many of the products on grocery shelves contain lots of salt, sugar, and fat added in processing. Luckily we're in an age where more and more manufacturers are listening to consumers, and making products that are far less fattening and refined. Keep your eyes open to what's happening in your grocery store; things are changing on a daily basis. Here are some highlights in each of the food sections to give you an idea of what's happening and what to look for.

PYRAMID FINDS IN THE FROZEN FOODS AISLE

Once upon a time frozen entrées, dinners, and side dishes were notorious for being especially high in sodium, fat, and cholesterol. Desserts that were less than pure fat and sugar were few and far between. Not so today. There are lots of good-tasting foods in the freezer case that are low in fat, cholesterol, and sodium. Many are tailor-made to fit the U.S. Dietary Guidelines and say so right on the package. Here are some of the particulars.

Years ago Stouffer's **Lean Cuisine** line set the standard for calorie-controlled entrées, with fewer than 300 calories per serving. This line of foods was probably the first attempt to meet the need for frozen entrées that were of good quality, tasty, and convenient, and had far fewer calories than had previously been available. Most of the entrées were, however, high in sodium. That's no longer the case since the entire line was reformulated. Each item has no more than 30 percent of calories from fat, no more than 65 milligrams of cholesterol, fewer than 600 milligrams of sodium, and less than 300 calories; canola is now the oil that is used for all Lean Cuisine entrées (changed from corn oil). The reduced amounts of fat, sodium, and cholesterol mean that the Lean Cuisine line fits right in with the Dietary Guidelines, and all the relevant information is clearly printed on the package. Several meatless entrées are also included to suit all preferences.

Smart Ones frozen entrées from the Weight Watchers Food Company are all made to have 1 gram of fat or less per entrée. They contain on average about 170 calories (with a range of 120 to 220 per entrée) and 400 milligrams of sodium each. None of the entrées contains more than 60 milligrams of cholesterol. Ethnic choices provide for a wide range of tastes and flavors, which include Shrimp Marinara with Linguine, Chicken Français, Pasta Portofino, and Fiesta Chicken.

Weight Watchers also knows that busy Americans often want a nutritious breakfast but rarely have the time to prepare it. **Weight Watchers Breakfast On The Go!** fills that need. Each item is hand-held and meant to be portable. The choices include Garden Omelet Sandwich, Blueberry Muffins, Banana Nut Muffins, and a Ham and Cheese Bagel.

Healthy Choice is a full line of breakfasts, dinners, entrées, French bread pizzas, breaded fish items, and dairy desserts. They even offer some canned foods and spaghetti sauces. When the president of ConAgra foods had his own personal heart-health problems, the foods were developed for anyone who wanted to make healthier choices in frozen prepared foods. Healthy Choice also adheres to the Dietary Guidelines for less fat, cholesterol, and sodium. Items like Western-Style Omelet on English Muffin, Rigatoni with Chicken, Beef Enchilada, Lemon Pepper Fish, and Old-Fashioned Vanilla frozen dessert appeal to every palate imaginable. Each of the packages gives the full nutrition analysis in a clear, easy-to-read format.

▲▲

FROZEN FOOD TIPS

▲ Choose low-fat or nonfat frozen yogurts and nondairy desserts; look for frozen fruit or juice bars without added sugar.

▲ Buy preportioned cups, bars, and cones to help you resist eating more than you want to.

▲ Look for frozen fudge bars made with dry skim milk. They can be under 100 calories per bar and provide extra calcium.

▲ Team up frozen meals with a stop at the salad bar for a side salad, some breadsticks, and fruit to round out the meal.

▲ Buy frozen vegetables packed in large bags for the sake of economy, and for the comfort of knowing there is always enough for one person or for six.

▲ Select interesting frozen vegetable medleys and ethnic combinations (Japanese, Mediterranean, or Mexican varieties); they're ready-to-use and save you lots of peeling and prep time.

▲ Frozen fruit juice concentrates are often the least expensive form of juice; thawed and undiluted they also make a nice sweetener to use instead of sugar.

▲ Frozen berries are often packed without extra sugar and when out of season are less expensive than fresh berries.

▲ Freeze your own cut-up fresh fruit for use throughout the year.

▲ Buy foods with "extras" like sauces, gravies, batters, breadings, etc., only occasionally. They add lots of sodium and fat to your daily intake.

▲ Read the labels for the final word. They give the real information on how "light," or "healthy" a product really is.

▲ Keep your freezer at 0° F. Use a thermometer to be sure.

▲▲

The acclaimed Canyon Ranch Spas have developed a full line of meals that can be delivered to your home or office simply by dialing 800-84-RANCH. Some specialty and gourmet stores are also carrying the food, which is high in complex carbohydrates and fiber, but low in fat, cholesterol, sugar, and sodium. The meals are actually refrigerated and can be heated in a few minutes by microwave, or in a regular oven. Registered dietitians are available to help you select menus based on your needs, if you like. The wide range of selections includes Raisin Sourdough French Toast, Country Lentil Soup, Shrimp with Sweet and Sour Sauce, Vegetarian Chili, Chicken Provençal, Lasagna Florentine, Salmon Tarragon, Raisin Oatmeal, and Raspberry Fruit Center Cookies (from Healthy Valley).

Frozen fruits and vegetables are smart foods to keep on hand. Some of your favorite produce items may not be in season all year long, or may be very expensive out of season. Frozen foods can guarantee your getting the recommended five servings of good-tasting fruits and vegetables any time your heart desires. The quality of these frozen items has improved tremendously over the years. I especially like the plastic bags of assorted vegetables and fruits that don't have any added fats or salt. They can be used in any number of ways.

Also check the freezer case for frozen breads and pizza dough, as well as a wide assortment of baked muffins, cakes, and desserts. Many of them are made with little or no fat, and are quite delicious. The advent of Simplesse, an all-natural fat substitute, has certainly changed the profile of frozen desserts. Not only is Simplesse a fat-free replacement, it also offers a creamy, rich texture to the foods in which it is used. Simple Pleasures frozen dessert was the first product on the market made with Simplesse, which has a wide variety of uses in foods including salad dressings, baked goods, dips, puddings, cheeses, and margarine.

PYRAMID PICKS
IN THE PRODUCE SECTION

Just about every item in the produce section is a Pyramid-style food. Fresh fruits and vegetables are high in vitamins, minerals, and fiber. Best of all they are low in fat, calories, and sodium. (Coconuts, avocados, and nuts, though, are the few items that do contain fat, so choose them more moderately.)

Many supermarkets have salad bars that make it easy to work in our daily servings of fruits and vegetables. When I have guests at the last minute, or am really pressed for time, I buy items from the salad bar like carrots, celery, spinach, mushrooms, strawberries, melon, and pineapple that are already washed, cut, and ready to use. It's a real treat to be able to pick up prepared ingredients for a stir-fry or a fruit salad. Although it is more expensive, the convenience is sometimes worth it. Do beware of some of the salad dressings, or toppings such as cheese, nuts, or bacon bits, which add heavily to the fat category. Some of the prepared salads like coleslaw, potato salad, and macaroni salad can also contain lots of fat and sodium.

PYRAMID PICKS IN THE DAIRY CASE

Our best sources of calcium are dairy products. They also provide a fair amount of protein and other valuable nutrients. But you must be careful—you can also bring home a lot of fat and sodium in dairy products. Check the labels to find out which ones are low in fat or completely fat-free.

Yogurts, for instance, come in a variety of styles, ranging from those made with skim milk to others made with whole milk and cream. Adding your own fruit to plain yogurt is the best way to reduce added sugar. You can also drain yogurts (see pages 64–70) to make thick, creamy cheeses, sauces, and toppings. Sour cream, too, has been trimmed down. Thanks to Simplesse, Light 'n Lively Light Sour Cream contains half the fat of regular full-fat sour cream and one-third fewer calories. It works well in salad dressings and in recipes that call for yogurt and mayonnaise.

Part-skim and nonfat natural cheeses are available in a wide variety. Some, however, leave a bit to be desired in the taste department; and most don't melt very well without drying out and turning to cardboard. The trick is to use them in casseroles or lasagnas, where there is moisture from other ingredients to maintain the texture of the cheese. Alpine Lace has some excellent nonfat cheeses, and Polly-O has done a nice job reducing—and even eliminating—the fat in some of the Italian cheeses like mozzarella and ricotta. Even some of the process cheeses like Velveeta are getting around to lowering their fat content, though most remain pretty high in sodium. You needn't eliminate any cheeses or dairy products because of their fat or sodium content. Remember to read the labels and know what you're buying. Then decide how much to buy and how often you'll eat certain foods.

PYRAMID PICKS AT THE MEAT COUNTER

Meat, poultry, game, and fish are all good sources of vitamins and minerals, and concentrated sources of protein. The fat content, however, varies widely. Sometimes it's hard to determine how much fat is in meat because many cuts contain fat in the muscle, or it is ground into chopped meat, making it hard to know the fat content. There are some ways to solve that dilemma. The sidebar below will help you with some solutions. Remember that processed meats like hotdogs, bacon, sausage, and luncheon meats tend to be high in sodium and fat. Even the so-called low-fat versions can contain a high number of fat calories. Look at the numbers and read the labels carefully to know what you're buying.

Consider some of the game meats, like venison, rabbit, and quail, that are making their way into butcher shops and many supermarkets. Ask your butcher to order some of these products if you don't see them in the case.

Shellfish is back on the list for smart shoppers. Though it contains cholesterol, shellfish does not raise blood cholesterol levels as was once thought because of certain unsaturated fatty acids that it contains. Some canned fish, like sardines and salmon, have soft, edible bones that can add significantly to our calcium quota. Look for canned fish that is packed in water, but note that some sardines packed in tomato sauce are lower in fat than those packed in water.

▲▲▲

LEAN CHOICES AT THE MEAT COUNTER

▲ Look at labels in the meat case too. *Regular, lean,* and *extra-lean* indicates the fat content, which varies from about 28 to 16 percent by weight.

▲ Grading can give you some idea of the fat content of beef. *Select*-grade beef contains less fat than *choice*, which contains less fat than *prime*.

▲ Trim visible fat, and add little or no fat during cooking to keep lean meat lean.

▲ Read labels on hotdogs, sausage, and luncheon meats. All tend to be high in fat and sodium. Some lean, low-fat, and low-sodium varieties are available.

▲ Look for nutrition labeling on poultry items.

▲▲▲

PYRAMID PICKS FOR PACKAGED FOODS

Convenience is what everyone is looking for. Every home cook uses canned and packaged foods to some degree or another. Some purists decry these foods loudly, but few can truly live without them. No argument that many of them are high in sugar, fat, and sodium, but like everything else there are much better choices available today than we had several years ago.

No-salt-added, reduced-sodium, and low-sodium products, low-fat, nonfat, and even reduced-sugar foods mean that you can make Pyramid-style selections and still keep convenience in the kitchen. It's a pleasure to see that even many snack-food companies are attending to health in new or modified products they sell. Pepperidge Farm markets its Low-Sodium Symphony Cracker Assortment for those concerned about extra salt. And the Wholesome Choice cookie line offers six varieties of cookies that all have 2 grams or less of fat and 60 to 70 calories each. These two products joined the Golden and Chocolate 98% Fat Free Pound Cakes that are also low in sodium and contain 1 gram or less of total fat.

Guiltless Gourmet has a wonderful line of Mexican snack foods that passes every flavor test you can imagine. I've served their mild and spicy bean dips, salsas, and Cheddar queso dips to rave reviews. All are fat-free, and the tortilla chips are baked—not fried—so they are cholesterol-free and contain very little fat. Though Guiltless Gourmet products started out in health food stores, they are beginning to find their way into supermarkets.

Nabisco reformulated the familiar Fig Newton to be totally fat-free and added apple and cranberry versions while they were at it. The SnackWell line of fat-free and reduced-fat cookies and crackers offers shoppers new options in many of the most popular snack varieties. The brand features chocolate chip cookies, cheese crackers, and cinnamon graham snacks.

If it's cakes and cookies you crave, Entenmann's has a line of baked goods that are fat-free and cholesterol-free, with less than 100 calories per serving in their coffee cakes or cookies. For those with less of a sweet tooth, popcorn can sometimes be a healthy snack. Most of the packaged microwave popcorn has had its fat reduced, making it a better choice than before. But for my money the best invest-ment is a microwave corn popper (or an electric corn popper) so that you can pop the kernels without any fat at all and control how much salt, if any, you add. If you are buying popcorn already popped, beware of packages hailing "no-cholesterol." That doesn't mean no fat, it only indicates vegetable oil (which doesn't contain cholesterol) was used, and the popcorn may actually be higher in total fat than other brands.

Whole grains, cereals, and breads are at the base of the Pyramid, and there's a lot to help you fill that quota in the packaged-food category. Check the grain section for new quick-cooking varieties of rice and barley or aromatic rices like Basmati and jasmine rice. Pasta comes in a wide variety of sizes and shapes to make eating it fun, even if you make it seven nights a week. If you have a gluten allergy try rice noodles, or other grains, which are gluten-free. Also look for the Ener-G line of foods for various allergy diets. (See page 227, for mail-order information).

Consider making your own muffins and cakes from mixes that have reduced or eliminated fat from the ingredients. Check cereal boxes for those that have less sugar. Many granola cereals are sweetened with fruit juices instead of sugar and come with no fat. Kellogg's has put the Food Pyramid with some meal-planning tips on two of its cereal boxes to show how cereals fit into the new guidelines. Remember that instant cereals in individual serving packets are much higher in sodium than regular and quick-cooking cereal. Read the label to check the fiber content as well. Get the most from your food dollar by choosing foods with less fat and sugar, and more fiber.

Many oils, salad dressings, mayonnaises, butters, and margarines are coming out in slimmer versions. Salad dressing and mayonnaise are both available in reduced-calorie or fat-free varieties. Kraft Free Nonfat Dressings offer several good-tasting, fat-free, cholesterol-free salad dressings. Depending on the flavor, they contain 6 to 20 calories per tablespoon. When you are making the transition to lower fat by making dressings or sauces from scratch, it's a good idea to start by mixing some full-fat mayonnaise with nonfat yogurt so there isn't a dramatic flavor loss. Gradual, permanent changes are much better than those that start out with gusto but are abandoned because the new version lacks taste or is otherwise disappointing.

GETTING THE FINAL WORD

With all the new foods, ingredients, and thousands of choices that are found on supermarket shelves, it's hard for any of us to stay informed about all the options.

▲▲

SNACK ATTACKS CAN BE SAFE

Check out the snack-food aisle for new or reformulated snacks that make for pretty good munching.

▲ Low- or no-cholesterol claims on popcorn packages may only mean that vegetable oil is used, so the popcorn may still be high in fat.

▲ Use a hot-air popper at home for a high-fiber, no-fat snack.

▲ Choose crackers and cookies that are lower in fat and sodium like rice cakes, crispbreads, matzoh, graham crackers, and gingersnaps.

▲ Look for cookies made with whole-grain flour, oatmeal, dates, raisins, or figs, which provide more fiber than other cookies. Many of these kinds of cookies are now even made in fat-free forms.

▲ Eat pretzels for lower-fat and -sodium snacks; even salted pretzels are lower in salt than many other salty snacks.

▲ Carry small boxes of raisins for a quick, portable snack.

▲▲

What you read on the label should always be the last word in helping you make a savvy food choice. Labels give you ingredient information and nutrition information, as well as open dating (freshness information). Reading labels can help you choose foods that are lower in sugars, sodium, and fat. Reading labels can help you build a Pyramid of your own every time you go to the supermarket.

▲▲

PYRAMID EATING WHEREVER YOU GO

FAST FOOD

Sure you can eat at your favorite fast-food restaurant and still be within the Food Guide Pyramid. But selecting a nutritious meal at quick service restaurants can sometimes be a challenge. All it takes is some awareness of what you are ordering and a little planning. There is no question that quick service restaurants today are part of the American life-style. These restaurants keep customers coming back because they are fast, convenient, and the foods they serve are familiar and consistent no matter where in the world you eat them.

Foods served in quick service restaurants tend to be low in fiber, high in sodium, and provide a lot of calories from fat, particularly saturated fat. We should remember that when most of these restaurants started, that's how most Americans ate: meat and potatoes were the basis of our diet. Over the years evidence emerged about the relationship of diet and health with recommendations for different eating patterns. Many of the quick service menu boards have changed to reflect the new trends and consumer requests for foods with less fat, calories, and sodium. Many companies have broadened their menus to include new, healthy, and appealing choices. In response to the nutrition concerns of the consumer, and the demands for more nutrition information, many of the chains have developed dietary analyses of their food and beverage items. And most of them have printed this information in brochures that are available at the restaurant counter.

As in most other areas of the quick service business, McDonald's has taken the lead in the nutrition arena. McDonald's was the first to post nutrition and ingredient information of all their menu items; posters are displayed in the lobby of all U.S. restaurants as a quick guide to the healthiest choices. Customers can see at a glance the nutrition analysis of each item, and know how each fits into their daily meal plan.

Try to make choices at quick service restaurants the same way you make choices at any other time during the day. Keep in mind variety, balance, and moderation, the backbone of the Food Guide Pyramid. With these concepts it is possible—and permissible—to enjoy quick service restaurant meals. Choose foods from each of the layers, or food groups, of the Pyramid. Remember that no one food supplies all of the protein, vitamins, and minerals you need for good health. You can incorporate variety with food selections you make throughout the entire day. Vary choices wherever you go. In a quick service restaurant have a soft drink one time and low-fat milk the next. Order fries on one visit, a salad on the next.

Balance what you're ordering at a fast-food restaurant with what you've had—or are going to have—the rest of the day. You really can have just about whatever you want—even if you make the higher-fat choices—when you balance out the other meals of the day. For instance, if you've decided that nothing can replace your favorite deluxe burger with the works, then simply fit it into your eating agenda for the day. To accommodate that burger and fries, choose a lower-fat breakfast, like a bagel, or fat-free yogurt, or cereal and skim milk; and for dinner have some poached fish with lots of vegetables, or perhaps rice or pasta and a light sauce, with some fresh fruit for dessert.

It's all a matter of *planning* your menu selections. The key to maintaining a healthier life-style and enjoying your fast-food favorites is easy once you are familiar with the nutrient content of the foods and how they relate to your goals. Determine your personal daily fat-gram target as suggested earlier (see page 37), and then spread your fat allowance accordingly over the foods you eat in a day. It is also important to be flexible in controlling your fat grams; your target is only an average and may be higher some days and lower on others. Request nutrition information to make planning easier (see page 212).

Eating nutritious meals-on-the-run may be a challenge, but it's hardly impossible. Look below for a sample of the more nutritious selections available at several of the major quick service restaurants. Be creative with fast-food fare, choose the items that you like, and always feel free to make special requests.

McDonald's

Since 1973, McDonald's has provided nutrition information to consumers, and over the years has developed a number of more healthful menu options. Today the wallet cards with the information for "Food Exchanges" and "Calorie, Fat, Cholesterol, and Sodium" are available in most restaurants. McDonald's has also made a lot of behind-the-scenes changes: they have reformulated, or added, menu items that are more nutritious *and* taste delicious.

In 1983 they reduced the sodium in breakfast sausages by 32 percent, in 1984 the sodium in the pickles was reduced by 21 percent, and in 1987 the sodium in the pancakes was reduced by 30 percent. All buns are fortified with calcium, as are the English muffins. Fresh salads were introduced in 1986, and only 100 percent vegetable oil is used for cooking. Few people realize that the frozen yogurt served is 99 percent fat-free, and that all milk is 1% low-fat milk. Whole-grain cereals and fat-free, cholesterol-free apple-bran muffins were added to the breakfast menu. Fat in both the Big Mac and tartar sauce has been reduced (lowering the calories in the Big Mac and Filet-O-Fish sandwiches). Margarine replaced butter in all McDonald's restaurants, and both the fat and calories have been reduced in all salad dressings. Shredded carrots, not shredded cheese, is used on some salads. And burger history was made in 1991 with the introduction of the McLean Deluxe, which is 91 percent fat-free and contains just 10 grams of fat.

Anyone can request a copy of "McDonald's: Food the Facts," which includes complete nutrition and ingredient nutrition for all standard menu items. A series of "Did You Know?" leaflets, available in each restaurant, covers areas of interest to customers from nutrition to the environment.

McDonald's has always supported and promoted educating the consumer on how to eat out the Dietary Guidelines way. The Food Guide Pyramid was the center of a series of nutrition public service announcements developed in partnership with the Society for Nutrition Education for Saturday mornings on CBS. "What's on Your Plate" featured Willie Munchright and friends teaching kids about foods and how to make healthy food choices. The announcements were turned into a teaching kit distributed to teachers and health professionals with a videocassette, leader's guide, and an activity brochure that included the Food Pyramid. The Pyramid theme was also carried over to another campaign that McDonald's developed in partnership with the American Dietetic Association, called Food FUNdamentals. Included in the Happy Meal, this program was also specifically designed to complement the Food Guide Pyramid. It consisted of a series of toy food characters and nutrition activity pamphlets that featured games and riddles to help children learn about the food groups, and what it means to eat in a healthful way. It was a special promotion for National Health Month in 1992.

MAKE-THE-RIGHT-CHOICE SAMPLE MENUS:

Breakfast

Whole-Grain Cereal (Wheaties or Cheerios)*
1% Lowfat Milk, 8 fl. oz.
Orange Juice, 6 fl. oz.

270 calories ▲ 3 grams fat ▲ 10 mg cholesterol ▲ 340 mg sodium

* If you substitute McDonald's Fat Free Apple Bran Muffin for the cereal,

370 calories ▲ 2 grams fat ▲ 10 mg cholesterol ▲ 330 mg sodium

Scrambled Eggs
English Muffin
Orange Juice, 6 fl. oz.

390 calories ▲ 14 grams fat ▲ 425 mg cholesterol ▲ 560 mg sodium

Lunch/Dinner

Chunky Chicken Salad
Lite Vinaigrette Dressing, 1 pkt.
Iced Tea, medium

198 calories ▲ 6 grams fat ▲ 78 mg cholesterol ▲ 470 mg sodium

McLean Deluxe
Side Salad, Lite Vinaigrette Dressing, ½ pkt.
Diet Coke, small

375 calories ▲ 12 grams fat ▲ 93 mg cholesterol ▲ 845 mg sodium

Chicken Fajita, 1 (available at participating McDonald's)
Vanilla Lowfat Frozen Yogurt Cone
Diet Coke, medium

297 calories ▲ 9 grams fat ▲ 38 mg cholesterol ▲ 415 mg sodium

Jack in the Box

Jack in the Box has recently revised its brochure, which now provides complete nutritional information for menu items. This includes suggested meal combinations and some "good health tips" like: Learn More About Your Body; Maintain a Healthy Weight; Eat Regular Meals; Eat Plenty of Grain Products, Fruits and Vegetables; and Aim for a Diet Low in Fat, Saturated Fat and Cholesterol. Other dietary tips are: Get to Know Your Diet Pitfalls; Reduce Don't Eliminate Certain Foods; Make Changes (in Eating Habits) Gradually; and Balance Food Choices Over Time. The brochure also gives a graphic of the Food Guide Pyramid and the number of servings suggested in each food group.

MAKE-THE-RIGHT-CHOICE SAMPLE MENUS

Breakfast

Breakfast Jack
Orange Juice, 6.5 ounces

490 calories ▲ 13 grams fat ▲ 203 mg cholesterol ▲ 871 mg sodium

Sourdough Breakfast Sandwich
Orange Juice, 6.5 ounces

564 calories ▲ 20 grams fat ▲ 236 mg cholesterol ▲ 1,120 mg sodium

Lunch/Dinner

Hamburger
Side Salad, Low-Calorie Italian Dressing,* 70 grams
Diet Coke, small

344 calories ▲ 16 grams fat ▲ 26 mg cholesterol ▲ 1,485 mg sodium

* Not for those watching sodium; 1 serving has 810 mg (one-third of the daily recommended sodium).

Chef Salad
Diet Coke, small

325 calories ▲ 18 grams fat ▲ 142 mg cholesterol ▲ 900 mg sodium

Chicken Fajita Pita
Diet Coke, small

293 calories ▲ 8 grams fat ▲ 34 mg cholesterol ▲ 738 mg sodium

Wendy's

Wendy's was the first in the fast-food industry to introduce baked potatoes and the salad bar nationwide. Wendy's has a wide variety of lower-fat food choices. Among them are Wendy's Grilled Chicken Sandwich, Chili, and a variety of fresh Salads to Go, and Wendy's Garden Spot Salad Bar, which includes a host of fresh vegetables. When a reduced-calorie dressing is selected and paired with a plain baked potato, it can provide a well-balanced, low-fat, nutritious meal. Just as in other quick service restaurants, you need to watch out for high-fat dressings and toppings that can add a lot of calories, fat, and sodium. For example, 2 tablespoons of the Italian Caesar Salad Dressing provides 150 calories, 16 grams fat, and 260 mg sodium; and two tablespoons of the Blue Cheese Dressing provides 180 calories, 19 grams fat, and 200 mg sodium. Try topping your salad instead with 2 tablespoons of Wendy's Reduced Calorie Italian Dressing, which provides only 50 calories and 4 grams fat, but does have 340 mg sodium. If sodium is a concern, try pairing 1 tablespoon of Salad Oil (120 calories, 14 grams fat, no sodium), and 1 tablespoon Wine Vinegar (2 calories, less than 1 gram fat, and only a trace of sodium). Beware of Wendy's Superbars (Mexican Fiesta or Pasta Bar), which are loaded with prepared salads that contain a lot of mayonnaise and oily dressings, like potato salad, macaroni salad, and coleslaw.

Lunch/Dinner

Grilled Chicken Sandwich
Side Salad with Reduced Calorie Dressing
Lemonade

500 calories ▲ 14 grams fat ▲ 60 mg cholesterol ▲ 1,210 mg sodium

Small Chili, 9 oz.
Side Salad with Reduced Calorie Dressing
Iced Tea

250 calories ▲ 9 grams fat ▲ 40 mg cholesterol ▲ 870 mg sodium

Fresh Salad to Go

Deluxe Garden Salad with Reduced Calorie Dressing
Baked Potato
Diet Coke, small

461 calories ▲ 9 grams fat ▲ no cholesterol ▲ 750 mg sodium

Hardee's and Burger King

Hardee's offers breakfast and lunch/dinner selections that are lower in fat and calories. Three Pancakes are a lower-fat and lower-calorie breakfast option. Healthier options at lunch and dinner include the Regular Roast Beef Sandwich, Grilled Chicken Breast Sandwich, and the Garden Salad. With careful planning, a few choices can also be made at Burger King. While some of these meals may be low-calorie and low-fat, they can be quite high in sodium. For example, the BK Broiler Chicken Sandwich provides 280 calories, 10 grams fat, and 770 mg sodium. The Chunky Chicken Salad is a better choice, providing 142 calories, 4 grams fat, and 443 mg sodium. If sodium is a concern, request that salt be omitted from the preparation or limit your visits. Sodium here is hard to avoid.

HARDEE'S

Breakfast

Three Pancakes
1% Lowfat Milk
Orange Juice

530 calories ▲ 4 grams fat ▲ 25 mg cholesterol ▲ 1,025 mg sodium

Lunch/Dinner

Grilled Chicken Breast Sandwich
Side Salad with Fat-Free Dressing
Diet Coke, medium

331 calories ▲ 9 grams fat ▲ 60 mg cholesterol ▲ 905 mg sodium

Hamburger
Garden Salad with Fat-Free French Dressing
Diet Coke, medium

445 calories ▲ 22 grams fat ▲ 64 mg cholesterol ▲ 760 mg sodium

BURGER KING

Lunch/Dinner

BK Broiler Sandwich
Side Salad with Light Italian Dressing
Diet Coke, medium (22 ounces)

335 calories ▲ 11 grams fat ▲ 50 mg cholesterol ▲ 1,480 mg sodium

Chunky Chicken Salad with Light Italian Dressing
French Fries, medium (salted)
Orange Juice, 6.5 ounces

626 calories ▲ 25 grams fat ▲ 49 mg cholesterol ▲ 1,393 mg sodium

TIPS FOR EATING ON THE RUN

▲ Limit deep-fried foods such as fish and chicken sandwiches and chicken nuggets, which are often higher in fat than plain burgers. If you are having fried chicken, remove some of the breading before eating.

▲ Order roast beef, turkey, or grilled chicken, where available, for a lower-fat alternative to most burgers.

▲ Choose a small order of fries with your meal rather than a large one, and request no salt. Add a small amount of salt yourself if desired. If you are ordering a deep-fat-fried sandwich or one that is made with cheese and sauce, skip the fries altogether and try a plain baked potato (add butter and salt sparingly), or a dinner roll instead of a biscuit; or, try a side salad to accompany your meal instead.

▲ Choose regular sandwiches instead of "double," "jumbo," "deluxe," or "ultimate." And order plain types rather than those with "the works," such as cheese, bacon, mayonnaise, and "special" sauce. Pickles, mustard, ketchup, and other condiments are high in sodium. Choose lettuce, tomatoes, and onions.

▲ At the salad bar, load up on fresh greens, fruits, and vegetables. Be careful of salad dressings, added toppings, and creamy salads (potato salad, macaroni salad, coleslaw). These can quickly push calories and fat to the level of other menu items or higher.

▲ Many fast-food items contain large amounts of sodium from salt and other ingredients. Try to balance the rest of your day's sodium choices after a fast-food meal.

▲ Alternate water, low-fat milk, or skim milk with a soda or a shake.

▲ For dessert, or a "sweet-on-the-run," choose low-fat frozen yogurt where available.

▲ Remember to balance your fast-food choices with your food selections for the whole day.

▲▲▲

Trends show that an increasing number of people are eating in quick service restaurants, and they are also eating there on a more frequent basis because convenience and low prices are appealing in today's fast-paced society. Therefore, the impact of fast foods on our health and nutritional status can be a big one. Learning how to choose foods when eating out is more important than ever. It is possible to enjoy fast food the Pyramid way. You can have your burger—and eat it too.

In addition to obtaining nutrition information in brochures, consumers with questions can call the customer-service phone lines of most quick service restaurants. The following numbers are for customers with nutrition questions and general questions, queries, or comments: McDonald's (708) 575-FOOD, Wendy's (614) 764-6800, Hardee's (800) 346-2243, and Burger King (800) YES-1-800.

PYRAMID IN THE SKY

The nutritional status and quality of airplane meals has been gradually upgraded. This is a reflection of passengers' increased health concerns and their expectations for quality meals. In many cases, airplane fare is a well-balanced meal. Sometimes it provides at least one serving from most, if not all, of the food groups. In fact, serving sizes on airplanes can serve as a tool to teach us how to distinguish what an actual "serving size" is. If the standard meals don't suit you, or if you have religious or dietetic restrictions, the majority of airlines can accommodate these with their special meal programs.

Although you may think the portion size of airplane meals is quite small, the reality is that the tray before you will almost always contain one to two servings from each food group. One serving of meat (usually chicken or beef) on a typical tray is usually about 3 ounces, while the remaining sections on the tray most often contain about one to two servings from the Bread Group (one roll, and ½ cup pasta or rice), two servings from the Vegetable Group (1 cup tossed salad and ½ cup cooked vegetables), one serving from the Fruit Group (1 medium-size apple or ½ cup fruit cocktail), and depending on whether breakfast, lunch, or dinner is being served, one serving from the Milk, Yogurt, and Cheese Group (an 8-ounce carton of milk or yogurt, or 2 ounces of processed cheese). Additional servings from the food groups can be provided from the snacks (peanuts, pretzels, or fruit) and beverages (fruit or vegetable juice, milk, etc.), or perhaps an additional meal on longer flights.

Today most of the airlines realize that people make a conscious effort to maintain their diets even when flying. Sky Chefs, an airline catering company, has jumped on the better-nutrition bandwagon to satisfy preferences for lighter and healthier food. Pasta, poultry, fish, salads, and soups now stand alongside popular beef dishes. Olive oil and light sauces have replaced butter and cream sauces, tropical oils, and sugary glazes. Factory-made omelets and pancakes have been replaced by lighter breakfast menus that include low-fat yogurt, seasonal fruit salad, plain bagels, whole-grain cereals with skim milk, and no-yolk (no-cholesterol) omelets made with Egg Beaters. As requests for these kinds of meals increase, the variety of special meals expands, and airlines continue to revise their menus according to passenger preference studies.

Although some airlines offer more special meals than others, most of the special meal "categories" on the major airlines are the same. These include: Bland or Soft, Diabetic, Low-Carbohydrate, Gluten-Free, Lactose-Free, Low-Calorie, Low-Fat/Cholesterol, Low- or No-Sodium, Strict Vegetarian, Lacto-Ovo Vegetarian, Hindu, Muslim, Kosher, Child, Infant or Toddler, Fruit Plate, and a Fish or Seafood Plate. Some airlines offer unique special-order meals; for example, US Air offers a High-Protein meal, usually ordered by athletes. These are well-seasoned menus that include added dairy products and larger portions of meat and seafood to increase the protein. United Airlines' special meal program is currently undergoing expansion to include low-protein, low-purine, and high-fiber meals. Delta Airlines has nineteen special meals, including an Asian meal, available to its passengers.

To show you how the Food Pyramid is incorporated into menu planning, let's use United Airlines' low-calorie, low-sodium lunch or dinner. A sample menu includes a tossed salad, Weight Watchers salad dressing (optional); a wheat dinner roll, margarine (optional); Mrs. Dash (a sodium-free blend of herbs); a 4-ounce (cooked) steamed skinless chicken breast; Parsleyed Potatoes, Broccoli Florets, and Yellow Squash; and a fresh fruit dessert. All of the vegetables are prepared without added fat or salt. According to the Food Guide Pyramid, this meal provides one serving from the Bread Group, about three servings from the Vegetable Group, one serving from the Fruit Group (two servings if fruit juice is the beverage of choice), one-and-a-half servings from the Meat Group, and a minimal amount of fats and oils.

On US Air, a low-sodium or low-cholesterol meal might include: tossed salad, dietetic salad dressing (optional); a 4-ounce grilled chicken breast marinated in orange juice and sherry; steamed rice; steamed green vegetable; fresh fruit salad; small dinner roll or muffin and unsalted margarine (optional). Grains are being incorporated into more menus. The Vegetarian Menu might include a Vegetarian Barley Casserole, a Grain-and-Veggie Medley, a Yam-and-Apple Casserole made with oatmeal, or Baked Barley with Vegetables. Continental Airlines reports that its vegetarian menu is among the most preferred of their special meals. It includes Couscous with Corn and Celery, and a Chickpea–Kidney Bean Salad.

American Airlines is particularly dedicated to the health of its passengers. In addition to the sixteen special meals offered, American now offers low-cholesterol

"Heart Healthy Meals," developed in consultation with nutrition and medical experts at the Cooper Clinic Aerobics Center in Dallas, Texas. American has also teamed up with Weight Watchers Food Company to have their low-fat, low-calorie, low-cholesterol, and reduced-sodium entrées redesigned. The entrées are rotated every three months; two sample entrées are Chicken Fettucini (240 calories, 8 grams fat, 430 mg sodium, 15 mg cholesterol, and 21 grams carbohydrates), and Garden Lasagna (210 calories, 5 grams fat, 330 mg sodium, 10 mg cholesterol). All of the Weight Watchers entrées are accompanied by a tossed salad with Weight Watchers dressing, a multigrain roll with unsalted margarine, and fresh sliced fruit for dessert. A pamphlet that describes the entrée and gives a nutrient analysis of the meal is also included on the tray. The "American Traveler Menu" is unique to American Airlines. It offers fresh alternatives to the airlines' standard fare. Breakfast/Brunch menus on the American Traveler include fresh seasonal fruits, low-fat yogurt, low-fat cheese, and Egg Beaters. Lunches and dinners change on a monthly basis, and include entrées such as Poached Salmon with Carrots and Parsley Potatoes (February and April), Chilled Lime Ginger Chicken with Sugar Peas and Coleslaw (July), and Halibut Steak with Broccoli and Cornmeal Cake (November).

These special meal programs should be taken advantage of, as they are not only healthy alternatives, but the food often tastes better, too. Advance notice on the major airlines usually requires a minimum of six to eight hours (longer when ordering kosher meals), so be sure to plan ahead, or request your special meal when booking your flight.

THE FLOATING PYRAMID

A cruise vacation once meant dieting weeks before your trip, followed by some more dieting after your trip. Weight gain has always been a concern for cruise passengers. The elaborate and sumptuous buffets, with the overwhelming number of choices, made the temptation to load your plate with everything in sight easier than attempting to make healthy selections. Fortunately, even luxury liners have taken great steps to use the Pyramid recommendations and develop new and healthier menus. Chefs on cruise ships now offer delicious alternatives that allow you the pleasure of indulging, but without the guilt and gain. Today's luxury liners offer more fitness facilities and exercise classes, and some even have nutrition counseling available. The fitness programs are complemented by menus that include fresher, lighter, and more healthful options that are low in fat, calories, cholesterol, and sodium. While the Food Pyramid has not yet been directly incorporated into the menu planning aboard luxury liners, the lighter menus reflect today's awareness of the need for a healthy and well-balanced diet.

For those who might want to try to lose weight on a cruise vacation, or simply not gain weight, Cunard Cruises offers the Golden Door Spa at Sea program aboard four of its liners. Representatives from the famous Golden Door of Escondido, California, are aboard each ship, organizing daily fitness classes and offering individual consultation on diet and exercise. The menu provides Golden Door selections, each with the calorie count—including Chef's Suggestions and Golden Door Suggestions. Golden Door suggestions aboard Cunard's *Sea Goddess* include a Bibb Lettuce and Snow Pea Salad with Lemon Vinaigrette (70 calories), Brochette of Chicken and Spring Vegetables served over Couscous and Curried Flageolets (320 calories), and Poached Pear and Blackberry Purée (160 calories) for dessert. These dishes are part of a seven-day meal plan that is calculated to provide maximum energy during weight loss. As a passenger aboard the Cunard *Countess*, you can take advantage of the SeaSports program. This is a combination of sports and other activities on land and at sea, including supervised fitness training sessions. A dinner selection from the lighter SeaSports menu may include Seasonal Sliced Melon, consommé, Escalope of Veal-Picata, steamed baby carrots, baked potato, Romaine salad, and for dessert a selection of fresh fruit. For travelers aboard Cunard's luxurious *QE2*, a spa menu is offered alongside the regular menu, and a diabetic dessert (though not necessarily low-calorie) is always available along with the regular dessert selection.

The Royal Caribbean Cruise Line has developed the ShipShape Program, where exercise and healthy eating are both encouraged. Low-fat, low-cholesterol selections are available for every course on the menu as part of the ShipShape Program. A ShipShape menu may include: Ambrosia Fruit Cocktail appetizer, consommé, Heart of Lettuce Salad with Carrot Curls, Boston Sole served with Mushrooms, Green Peppercorn Sauce, Tomato Rockefeller, Red Bliss Potatoes and Broccoli Florets, and for dessert, lemon sherbet. Spaghetti with tomato sauce and fresh seasonal fruits are additional low-fat selections that are available nightly, along with the newest addition to the menu's sugar-free desserts. As for the future, Stephan Gras, corporate director of food operations for Royal Caribbean, says that there are plans to include low-sodium and gluten-free selections.

The Princess Cruise Line offers a program called Cruisercise, which includes exercise classes such as aerobics, walk-a-mile, and more. Low-fat, low-cholesterol, and low-sodium dishes are designated on the menu. Upon request, the chefs can accommodate personal requests, such as sautéing, grilling, or broiling instead of frying, or replacing a cream sauce with a lighter vegetable sauce. And with a two-week advance notice, more complicated or specific diet requests can be accommodated.

Remember, for every piece of fresh fruit there is a piece of marble cheesecake nearby, and for every run around the deck there is the temptation to lounge in the sun. With cruises more often than with other travel vacations, healthy life-style habits often drown as the ship leaves port. But with the diverse activities and lighter menu selections aboard most luxury liners, you may just find yourself leaving a cruise vacation feeling better (and lighter) than when you boarded.

HEALTHY HOTEL

Some of the finest cuisine in the United States is served in hotels. Although the Food Guide Pyramid has not yet been directly incorporated into hotel menus, several hotels have been offering heart-healthy menu options for years. These usually mean that dishes are low in sodium, fat, and cholesterol. Some hotels even offer nutrient analyses on the menu, and if the information is not printed on the menu, many will supply it upon request. One company that has specifically revised its menu with the Food Pyramid in mind is the Marriott Hotel Division. The Lobby Bistro, at the Los Angeles Airport, is an example of one of Marriott's existing nutrition-conscious hotel restaurants. The restaurant is devoted to healthy dining and health-conscious eating, listing the calories, saturated fat, sodium, and cholesterol on several menu items. The menu is designed to allow you to mix and match according to your own taste. For example, you can order mesquite broiled fish and select which type of fish you want—halibut, swordfish, trout, tuna, salmon, or sea bass. Then you choose from a list of low-fat, low-calorie, low-sodium sauces—tomato basil, lemon ginger, or teriyaki. The meal also comes with fresh vegetables, a trip to the salad bar, and your choice of pasta seasoned with basil, oregano, and saffron; basmati rice; or boiled potatoes.

The Light Selection café menu is Ritz-Carlton's nationwide program that offers low-fat, low-cholesterol options for health-conscious guests. Some Light Selection lunch entrées at the Buckhead Ritz-Carlton in Atlanta, Georgia, include Steamed Norwegian Salmon with Watercress Sauce, a Steamed or Sautéed Vegetable Plate with Wild Rice or Potatoes, Poached Chicken Breast with Stir-Fry Vegetables and Light Soy Sauce, or a Seasonal Fruit Plate with Cottage Cheese or Yogurt. Although not printed on the menus, nutrition breakdowns of the Light Selection dishes are available upon request.

Chef Stephen Viggiano at the Ritz-Carlton in Palm Beach says that his menus were prepared with guest requests in mind, and the Food Guide Pyramid is evident in many of the preferred items. "Although most of our guests are not yet familiar with the Pyramid, they are seeking lighter, healthier meals and focusing on the Pyramid by concentrating on pastas, fruits, and fresh fish." The hotel features fresh Florida fish and local produce. Two of the recipes that are most favored by guests are Warm Grilled Seafood Salad served with a Cucumber Ginger Vinaigrette and Grilled Grouper and Angel Hair Pasta served with Tomato Vinaigrette.

The trademark for Hilton Hotels low-calorie fare is "Fitness First." The regular menus provide a separate section for at least three heart-healthy (low-calorie, low-fat, and low-cholesterol) dishes on both the lunch and dinner menus. In addition to the Fitness First menu selections, fresh fruits and vegetables, decaffeinated beverages, whole-grain breads, margarine, low-cholesterol dressing, skim milk, and more are available daily. At the San Diego Resort Hilton, the Fitness First menu includes seasonal Fresh Fruits with Frozen Low-Fat Yogurt and Banana Nut Bread (200 calories), or Herb-Broiled Breast of Chicken on a Bed of Corn-Blackbean Salsa and Blue Cornmeal Tortillas (775 calories). The Fitness First options on the room-service breakfast menu at the Atlanta Airport Hilton are low-fat plain yogurt, with or without fresh fruit and granola, or fresh fruit and cottage cheese. In addition, upon request, many of the items on the regular menu can be specially prepared to reduce calories, sodium, and cholesterol. To maintain Hilton's high standards of well-balanced, nutritious fare, all chefs complete a one-week nutritional training program at the Culinary Institute of America, under the guidance of a registered dietitian. Some of the Hilton Hotels work with the American Heart Association and display AHA's heart symbol (♥) next to the heart-healthy dishes.

These hotels represent a few of the nationwide chains that offer healthy alternatives to their guests. Until a greater number of hotels offer healthier selections, it is up to you, the guest, to order wisely from the menu. It is also up to you to inquire about cooking methods, portion size, and when necessary, to make special requests (see "Menu Literacy," page 221). Most hotel chefs will gladly honor your requests. This will help send out the message that your request is not just a "diet," or a trend, but a life-style.

PYRAMID RESTAURANT CUISINE

Today's chefs are reinventing the meal, just as the USDA reinvented the Food Wheel. Prominent chefs and restaurateurs all across the country are joining the Food Pyramid campaign to create dishes that are low in sodium, fats, and cholesterol. These chefs have responded to consumers' new appetite for food that is delicious as well as healthy and have incorporated a more balanced way of eating into their own diets. Chef/Proprietor Michael Foley, of Printers' Row and Le Perroquet in Chicago, is a chef who has created a menu for his customers that reflects his personal style of eating. "I don't want to serve my customers food that I wouldn't want to eat myself," says Foley. Chef/Proprietor Emeril Lagasse, of Emeril's and NOLA in New Orleans, improved his own diet by working one-on-one with a personal dietitian for about eight years. He has adapted a personal diet that stresses flavor, balance, and nutritional value.

Many chefs have reduced the portion size of the protein, and are serving larger portions of grains and pastas. Chefs now demonstrate creative ways to offer healthy dishes without sacrificing taste by saturating dishes with flavor, not fat, and by using more fresh herbs, not salt. While not all restaurants are officially designating menus as "Pyramid Cuisine," many have gone to great lengths to use fresher, often organic ingredients, and to develop new and healthier preparations. Here are some examples of what restaurants around the country are doing to prepare Pyramid-inspired food.

Leading the healthy life-style approach to eating is restaurateur Michael Franks, owner of four restaurants in the Los Angeles area: Chez Mélange in Redondo Beach, and Depot, Misto Caffe, and Fino, all in Torrance, California. Each of these restaurants offers a daily "Pyramid Plate" on its menu that adheres to the Food Guide Pyramid by being low-calorie, low-fat, and low-sodium. The calorie, fat, and cholesterol contents of these meals are listed on the menus. The emphasis of these Pyramid dinners is on carbohydrates, and all of these meals derive less than 30 percent of their calories from fat. At Depot, Franks designates the heart-healthy selections on this Cal-Asian-Mediterranean menu as "Heartistic Cuisine," while the low-fat selections served at Misto Caffe are described at "Heart Smart Cooking." At Chez Mélange, the heart-healthy dish of the day is referred to as the "Pyramid Plate," and is actually distinguished by a symbol for the Pyramid (▲) alongside the description of the dish on the menu. While it changes daily, the Pyramid meal might be Seared Pacific Albacore Tuna over Steamed Greens with Japanese Salsa, Basmati Rice, and Vegetables (300 calories, 5.5 grams fat, 52 mg cholesterol), or Seared Chilean Sea Bass over Steamed Oriental Greens with Yellow Thai Curry Yogurt Sauce, Basmati Rice, and Vegetables. Once every eight weeks at Chez Mélange is "Pyramid Night"—an extravaganza where ten Pyramid dishes are offered on the menu. Franks says that he believes in taking a "fun approach to eating healthy," and has plans to include Pyramid-shaped table tents explaining the USDA's Food Guide Pyramid.

In Chicago, diners out can eat healthy, fresh, and creative meals while following Pyramid guidelines. At Printers' Row, Chef/Proprietor Michael Foley refers to the newer low-calorie dishes as "simple pleasures." His approach is to "replace high-fat meat dishes with healthier items by balancing the fat flavor with herbs and spices." For example, Chef Foley prepares a two-inch-thick grilled or roasted eggplant steak with curried couscous, chopped salsa, and steamed or roasted vegetables for those customers who want to enjoy the flavor and texture of a steak without the fat and cholesterol. He also uses vegetable juices to enhance the flavor of menu items, rather than heavy, fatty sauces. Foley says, "I always take the Food Pyramid into consideration when developing menus, keeping the protein size in relation to the plate. I use a sensible, low-fat balance of vegetables along with starches and carbohydrates." At Foley's contemporary French restaurant, Le Perroquet, instead of using traditional butter and cream sauces that add fat and calories, he uses nonconventional cooking methods to create flavor: fresh vegetable and fruit purées, flavored oils, and herb coatings for meat and fish. For example, the menu offers Rabbit Flavored with Red Pepper and Basil.

Also in Chicago, Chef/Proprietor Charlie Trotter, of Charlie Trotter's restaurant, has a versatile menu that features perfectly balanced meals with lots of grains and vegetables and limits portion sizes to totals of about three ounces of meat. He is a proponent of using infused oils and vinaigrettes to create sauces that are full of flavor, are easier to digest, have fewer calories, and taste better. Trotter also uses vegetable broths and light meat and fish reductions to create flavorful sauces for the fresh, seasonal ingredients that are the heart of his cooking. Diners can choose from three dégustation (tasting) menus: The eight-course Vegetable Dégustation, the eight-course Grand Dégustation (choice of two main courses—fish or meat), or the Super Grand Dégustation, where Trotter uses his impromptu cooking style to spontaneously prepare twelve original courses. Upon request, Chef Trotter will create an all-fish dégustation or a special five-course dégustation as a lighter option or pretheater meal. While the menus change daily, selections on the Vegetable Dégustation have included Terrine of Roasted Eggplant and Zucchini with Saffron Oil, Red Bell Pepper Juice and Crispy Celery Root Napoleon, and Ragout of Sweet Potato, Legumes, Sweet Corn, and Leeks with Red-Wine-Infused Turnip Broth. Chef Trotter's method of cooking, and his use of the freshest ingredients available are what makes his patrons leave feeling fulfilled, rather than full.

In New York City, Chef Alan Harding of Nosmo King has been preparing his own version of Pyramid Cuisine since the restaurant opened in 1989. Now he actually calls it that. Owner Steve Frankel shares Harding's philosophy of serving hearty and healthy cuisine, which has been the inspiration behind the Nosmo King menu. The focus of the plates at Nosmo are grains, legumes, and vegetables, with smaller portions of fish or meat. One example of a Pyramid-inspired dish is the Swordfish Burrito Plate, a 4-ounce (uncooked weight) portion of lean, marinated swordfish wrapped in a whole-wheat tortilla shell with spaghetti squash, brown rice/quinoa pilaf, refried beans braised with cinnamon, and jicama-carrot-red-onion salad.

At Union Square Café in New York City, Chef Michael Romano has developed the "Earth and Turf" for those patrons who prefer a smaller portion of meat or fish, and larger portions of vegetables and grains, rather than a plate that focuses mainly on the protein (meat or fish). This Pyramid-inspired idea is a portion-controlled plate that includes five seasonal vegetable components, grains, and a 3-ounce (uncooked weight) portion of protein that might be a grilled rib lamb chop, marinated venison, or swordfish steak. Chef Romano uses a larger variety of grains than he has in the past to create lower-fat accompaniments to main courses. He has also listened to consumer preferences for more vegetarian dishes and added the Union Square Salad of grilled, steamed, roasted, and marinated vegetables. The Roast Vegetable Sandwich on Grilled Seven-Grain Bread with Garlicky Chick-pea Spread successfully replaced the once popular Bacon, Lettuce, and Tomato Sandwich.

▲▲

MENU LITERACY

The first thing to remember is that you are the customer, and it is permissible to make special requests. Restaurants may not be able to accommodate every request, but most will do their best to make reasonable changes or assist you in making a suitable choice. Here are some tips to keep in mind when dining out:

▲ Balance your choices. If you choose one dish that is higher in fat or sodium, balance the meal by choosing another that is lower.

▲ Plan ahead, and balance the remainder of your meals for the day.

▲ Resist the temptation to overload on bread (and especially the butter) that arrives when you are seated. You can request that the bread be served with the meal, and you can eat it without butter.

▲ Ask about preparations and ingredients. Order fish, chicken, or meat broiled without added fat. Ask if the vegetables are fresh or canned, and if they are served with sauce, butter, or cream. Whether for meat, vegetables, or salad, request sauce or dressing on the side, and use it sparingly.

▲ Ask about serving sizes. Many restaurants serve anywhere from 6- to 10-ounce servings of meat, fish, and poultry. Request a half-portion, or share a full one with your dining partner. Order an appetizer as your main course. These are often ample enough to serve as a meal.

▲ Be familiar with menu descriptions. *Breaded, fried, creamy, pan gravy, au gratin, scalloped*, and *rich* are all signals of higher-fat foods. *Poached, roasted, stir-fried*, and *steamed* are usually lower-fat selections. *Smoked, pickled, marinated, with soy sauce, mustard sauce*, and *Creole-style* usually signal high-sodium dishes.

▲ Read the menu completely. Pay attention to garnishes and accompaniments. Some restaurants will create an original main-course plate made up of an assortment of garnishes—like fruits or vegetables—if that appeals to you.

▲ Try ordering one course at a time rather than ordering all courses at the beginning and finishing everything, even though there is too much, and you're already full. Request a take-home bag and use leftovers for another meal.

▲ Request that salt be omitted during preparation, and then add it yourself if necessary.

▲ Ask for items that you do not see. Cream is usually offered with coffee, but low-fat milk or skim milk is usually available upon request. Light soups and fresh fruit are often staple items in the kitchen, even if they are not featured on the menu.

▲ Look for fresh fruit sorbets, poached fruits, or a simple plate of fresh seasonal fruit to top off your meal.

▲▲

Perhaps the most innovative addition to the tradition of southern cuisine is the introduction of "New Orleans Lite Cuisine" at Emeril's Restaurant in the Warehouse District of New Orleans. Chef/Proprietor Emeril Lagasse's philosophy is to keep the regional feel and flavor of New Orleans cuisine while preparing it in a lighter fashion that is "pure, clean, well-balanced, and nutritious." Chef Lagasse incorporated the Food Pyramid as a guide to create a well-balanced menu with healthy dishes that people can enjoy. "I believe in simple food that is nutritious, full of flavor and texture," he says. "People are getting used to a plate where the protein is smaller, and there are larger portions of grains and vegetables." The menu at Emeril's offers a 4-ounce (uncooked weight) portion of Albacore Tuna served on a bed of Home-made Sweet Potato Pasta drizzled with Spicy Ginger Oil, or a Vegetable Plate with fourteen to sixteen different vegetables (grilled, roasted, and sautéed) served on a bed of homemade vegetable pasta with herb-infused oil.

What seems to be common among all of these chefs is that their menus and styles of cooking reflect their personal eating habits. Many of the chefs also get advice from nutritionists to help create healthier dishes with a greater variety of foods from all of the food groups. They use the versatility of flavor-absorbing grains, such as quinoa, bulgur, barley, millet, and couscous to create new and interesting dishes that are naturally low in fat. Herb-infused oils and vinaigrettes, broths, and purées enhance the flavor of dishes and create sauces that have only a fraction of the calories that conventional sauces based on butter and cream had in the past. If you are watching sodium intake, a word of advice is in order: Request that salt be omitted during preparation. If necessary, you can add it at the table to suit your own taste.

Great strides have been taken by chefs to create flavorful, healthy, and nutritionally balanced meals that utilize fresh seasonal ingredients, while following the recommendations to minimize sodium, fats, oils, and sugars. Meals no longer have to be focused around meat, rich sauces, and fats. Grains, fruits, and vegetables play a major role in adding flavor and appeal to dining out. Take a look at Menu Literacy (page 221) for some tips on ordering. Remember that it is now possible to enjoy a healthy and nutritionally balanced meal in a fine-dining atmosphere.

▲▲▲▲▲▲▲▲▲▲▲▲▲▲▲▲▲▲▲▲▲▲▲▲▲▲▲▲▲▲▲▲▲▲▲▲▲▲

MENUS

An asterisk indicates a recipe included in this book.

Red Texas Grapefruit Sections
Baked Orange French Toast*

Pear Nectar
California Apricot Waffles*

Roasted Cod with Peppers, Onions, and New Potatoes*
Steamed Spinach
Hands-off Whole-Wheat Cornmeal Bread*
Apricot Torte* with Frozen Yogurt or Lemon Sherbet

Ginger-Steamed Fish*
Aromatic Asian Rice*
Mustard-Lime Broccoli*
Fresh Melon, Pineapple, and Kiwi

Greek Rabbit Stew*
Wide Ribbon Noodles
Sesame-Dressed Field Greens with Apples and Water Chestnuts*
Lemon Poppy Bundt Cake*

Saffron-scented Risotto with Portobello Mushrooms*
Spinach, Citrus, and Goat Cheese Salad*
Whole-Wheat Sourdough Bread
Glazed Apples and Raisins*

Vegetable Lo Mein*
Grilled Bangkok Beef Salad*
Steamed Chinese Buns*
Fresh Melon Cubes

Chilled Asparagus and Grape Salad*
Toreador Chicken*
Tropical Succotash Sauté*
Tomato Bread Pudding*
Orange Sorbet

Silky Sweet Potato and Apple Bisque*
Brochettes of Venison with Rosemary-Juniper Sauce*
Aromatic Asian Rice*
Steamed Asparagus Spears
Chocolate Angel Food Cake*

Sun-dried Tomato and Garlic Dip*
Italian Garlic Toasts*
Penne with Beans and Greens*
Tossed Salad with Honey-Dijon Dressing*
Mixed Berry Tart*

Swiss Chard Soup*
Savory Peppered Corn Muffins*
Raspberry Sorbet

No-Fat/No-Sweat Lasagna with Spinach and Lentils*
Red Leaf and Romaine Lettuce Salad
Sesame Breadsticks
Honeydew Melon and Berries

▲▲

RESOURCES

EQUIPMENT

Magafesa
Box 328
Prospect Heights, IL 60070
708-705-8700

True state-of-the-art pressure cookers available in 6- and 8-quart capacity. Triple seal means safe and fast cooking.

Really Creamy Yogurt Cheese Funnel
Millhopper Marketing
1110 N.W. Eighth Avenue
Gainesville, FL 32601
904-373-5800
Fax: 904-373-1488

A handy mesh funnel that turns yogurt into cheese. Two low-fat, low-cholesterol, low-calorie cookbooks available for separate purchase.

Steelon Nonstick Cookware
601 Gateway Boulevard, Suite 1150
South San Francisco, CA 94080
415-871-2444
Fax: 415-952-7412

Nonstick coated pots and pans with superior anodized surface. Excellent for no-fat cooking; even distribution of heat. No scouring or scrubbing; very easy to clean.

Vertical Roaster
Spanek, Inc.
P.O. Box 2190
Saratoga, CA 95070
408-446-3000

A unique "Eiffel Tower" metal-frame design cooks poultry about 30 percent faster than by conventional methods. Less fat and less salt are needed and results actually produce birds that are more tender, juicy, and easy to carve. Special skewer system can also be used for kebobs and chops.

Arrowhead Mills
110 S. Lawton
Hereford, TX 79045
806-364-0730

Over 75 percent of the grains, seeds, flours, nuts, beans, cereals, and mixes are asserted organic. Products are sold mainly in health food stores, but mail order is available on request.

Broken Arrow Ranch
Mike Hughes
104 Junction Highway
Ingram, TX 78025
800-962-4263
Fax: 210-367-4988

Mail order and retail sales of free-range venison and other wild game including antelope, wild boar, and wild lamb. No drugs or hormones used; animals drink only pure, natural spring water. Cooking instructions and nutrition information provided.

Canyon Ranch Meals
P.O. Box 1688-181
Pittsfield, MA 01202
800-84-RANCH

A full line of nutritionally balanced (refrigerated) meals that are delivered to home or office by overnight courier. Also available in some specialty and gourmet stores. Registered dietitians available for assistance.

Classic Country Rabbit Company
P.O. Box 1412
Hillsboro, OR 97123
800-821-7426
Fax: 503-693-1080

Classic is a USDA-inspected processor of rabbit meat that provides the largest selection

available of fresh and frozen portion-cut meat. They also sell whole rabbit and rabbit sausage. Rabbit is naturally lean and high in protein, iron, and vitamin B_{12}. It's also low in fat, cholesterol, calories, and sodium.

Coleman Natural Meats, Inc.
5140 Race Court
Denver, CO 80216
800-422-8866
Fax: 303-297-0426

Supplier of natural beef, a specialty item raised without antibiotics and growth hormones; organic beef, a natural food specialty item produced without antibiotics and growth hormones and fed organically grown feed, raised on farmland certified to be free of herbicides and pesticides for at least three years; and Coleman's Alpine Lamb. Brochure and recipes available.

Dakota Lean Meats, Inc.
136 West Tripp
Winner, SD 57580
800-727-5326

Supplier of beef that is lower in fat, cholesterol, and calories; animals are bred to be genetically lean and are raised without hormones or antibiotics. Tenderloin steaks and 93 percent lean ground beef patties available by mail. Call toll-free number above for information and orders.

Dean & DeLuca
560 Broadway
New York, NY 10012
800-221-7714

Carries one of the largest selection of "boutique" dried beans in the country. Their dried beans have all been harvested within the past year and are quicker cooking than other dried beans. Dean & DeLuca also sells and ships a full line of gourmet and specialty items including olive oils, vinegars, spices, coffees, and cookbooks.

Ener-G Foods, Inc.
5960 First Avenue, S.
P.O. Box 84487
Seattle, WA 98124-5787
800-331-5222

Specialty food items, mixes, and baked goods for various allergy diets. These include wheat-free, gluten-free, lactose-free mixes, and egg replacers. They also sell and ship vacuum-packed baked goods, soups, pastas, crackers, and other items suitable for allergy-restricted diets.

Frieda's Finest Produce
P.O. Box 58488
Los Angeles, CA 90058
800-421-9477
Fax: 213-741-9443

Frieda's distributes and ships a wide variety of specialty fruits, vegetables, herbs, and items like packaged crepes. Excellent full-color brochures are available with information on cooking techniques, recipes, etc. A mail-order catalogue is also available for "sampler" baskets and single-item shipping. This line of produce is well distributed, with the Frieda's label in many supermarkets and specialty stores around the country.

Guiltless Gourmet
3709 Promotory Drive, S.
Austin, TX 78744
512-443-4373

A full line of baked (no-oil) tortilla chips, bean dips, and cheese dips with no fat, and mild, medium, and hot picante dips. All are full-flavored, delicious snacks. Available in health food and specialty food stores, and some supermarkets.

King Arthur Flour
R.R. 2, Box 56
Norwich, VT 05055
800-827-6836

The full line of flours and grains has been expanded to include herbs, extracts, syrups, preserves, pans, and practically any other item bakers might need. Their lighter, sweeter Hard White Whole-Wheat Flour can be substituted for regular all-purpose flour in most any recipe, with little change in taste, texture, or appearance.

Ventra Packing Co.
373 Spencer Street
Syracuse, NY 13204
315-422-9277

Enrico's line of spaghetti sauces are low in fat and sodium; also a full line of salsa, enchilada sauce, and barbecue sauce. Sold in some stores or call to order.

The American Institute for Cancer Research Newsletter
Washington, DC 20069
800-843-8114

An easy-to-read newsletter published four times a year; includes up-to-date research information, recipes, consumer tips, and more. Call for details.

Diet, Nutrition, and Cancer Prevention
National Cancer Institute
Office of Cancer Communications
Building 31, Room 10A24
Bethesda, MD 20892
800-4-CANCER

This booklet describes how following the Dietary Guidelines may help to prevent cancer. Gives sample menus and ways to translate guidelines into food choices. Also gives list of fat and fiber in common foods. Write for a free copy and enclose a SASE.

Dietary Guidelines for Americans
Consumer Information Center
Pueblo, CO 81009
No toll-free number

If you wonder what they are and if they really exist, write for a free copy and enclose a SASE.

Eat More Fruits and Vegetables—Five a Day for Better Health
National Cancer Institute
Office of Cancer Communications
Building 31, Room 10A24
Bethesda, MD 20892
800-4-CANCER

A handy reference to put this program into action. Charts with best sources of vitamins A and C and dietary fiber. Write for a free copy and enclose a SASE.

The Food Guide Pyramid
Superintendent of Documents
Consumer Information Center
Department 159-Y
Pueblo, CO 81009

A 29-page booklet that introduced the Pyramid. Explains each layer, the number of servings, how to lower fat, sugar, and sodium in your diet. Check or money order for $1.00.

The Food Guide Pyramid . . . Beyond the Basic 4
Food Marketing Institute
800 Connecticut Avenue, N.W.
Washington, DC 20006

A shorter version that includes tips, serving-size information, and recommendations for various ages and activity levels. Check or money order for $.50 + SASE.

Kellogg Company
P.O. Box CAMB
Battle Creek, MI 49016
800-962-1413 (weekdays 8 A.M. to 5 P.M., EST)

Has brochures on product information and nutritive values; will also answer questions and receive comments.

National Center for Nutrition and Dietetics
The American Dietetic Association
216 West Jackson Boulevard
Chicago, IL 60606
800-366-1655

Registered dietitians are available to talk with callers Monday through Friday 10 A.M. to 5 P.M., EST; recorded nutrition information available twenty-four hours a day.

Supermarket Scoop
Supermarket Savvy
P.O. Box 7069
Reston, VA 22091
703-742-3364

Six eight-page issues of new food product information; product comparison charts; and brand-name product listings.

SUPERMARKET PROGRAMS

Many supermarkets are tying into the Food Pyramid and have information, booklets, or newsletters. Here are some of the most notable for you to contact.

Giant Foods, Inc.
P.O. Box 1804, Dept. 597
Washington, DC 20013
301-341-4365

Pyramid education through "Healthy Start . . . Food to Grow On." Targets parents and kids. "Eater's Almanac" publication also distributed to shoppers with food and nutrition information.

Price Chopper/Golub Corp.
501 Duanesbury Road
Schenectady, NY 12306
518-355-5000

Pyramid illustrated and other topics in "Eat Wise, Health Wise" booklet. Some in-store demos, cholesterol screenings, and registered dietitians to answer questions.

Safeway Stores
201 4th Street
Oakland, CA 94660
Cherryl H. Bell, R.D., M.S.
510-891-3452

A bi-monthly newsletter for a nominal subscription charge. Free monthly nutrition pamphlets also available.

Stop & Shop
P.O. Box 1942
Boston, MA 02105
617-770-8895

"Leaner Choice Guide to Low-Fat Shopping" booklet and program to help shoppers make lower-fat choices. Food guides for each department.

Wegmans
P.O. Box 844
Rochester, NY 14692
716-328-2550

Weekly product newspaper with nutrition articles. Food Pyramid on their private-label baked goods. Paper danglers in-store highlight Pyramid and "Food You Feel Good About" items.

▲▲▲

BIBLIOGRAPHY

Finn, Susan, and Linda Stern Kass. *The Real Life Nutrition Book*. New York: Penguin Books, 1992.

Gelles, Carol. *The Complete Whole Grain Cookbook*. New York: David I. Fine, Inc., 1989.

————. *Wholesome Harvest: Cooking with the New Four Food Groups—Grains, Beans, Fruits, and Vegetables*. New York: Little, Brown and Company, 1992.

Herbst, Sharon Tyler. *Food Lover's Companion*. Hauppauge, N.Y.: Barron's Educational Series, 1990.

Prevention Magazine, editors of. *The Healing Foods Cookbook*. Emmaus, Pa.: Rodale Press, 1991.

Sass, Lorna J. *Cooking Under Pressure*. New York: William Morrow and Company, 1989.

————. *Recipes from an Ecological Kitchen*. New York: William Morrow and Company, 1992.

Sunset Magazine, editors of. *Fresh Produce*. Palo Alto: Lane Publishing Co., 1987.

Tribole, Evelyn. *Eating on the Run*. Champaign, Ill.: Leisure Press, 1992.

Winick, Myron. *The Columbia Encyclopedia of Nutrition*. New York: Perigee Books, 1989.

▲▲

CHARTS

NUTRITIONAL VALUE OF PRODUCE

	Serving Size g	Serving Size oz.	Calories	Protein g	Carbo-hydrate g	Fat g	Sodium mg	Dietary Fiber g
Apple, 1 med.	154	5.5	80	0	18	1	0	5
Asparagus, 5 spears	93	3.5	18	2	2	0	0	2
Avocado, 1/3 med.	55	2	120	1	3	12	5	2
Banana, 1 med.	126	4.5	120	1	28	1	0	3
Bell pepper, 1 med.	148	5.5	25	1	5	1	0	2
Broccoli, 1 med. stalk	148	5.5	40	5	4	1	75	5
Cabbage, 1/12 med. head	84	3	18	1	3	0	30	2
Cantaloupe, 1/4 med.	134	5	50	1	11	0	35	0
Carrot, 1 med., 7" long, 1 1/4" diameter	78	3	40	1	8	1	40	1
Cauliflower, 1/6 med. head	99	3	18	2	3	0	45	2
Celery, 2 med. stalks	110	4	20	1	4	0	140	2
Cherries, 21 cherries; 1 cup	140	5	90	1	19	1	0	3
Cucumber, 1/3 med.	99	3.5	18	1	3	0	0	0
Grapes, 1 1/2 cups	138	5	85	1	24	0	3	2

	Serving Size g	Serving Size oz.	Calories	Protein g	Carbo-hydrate g	Fat g	Sodium mg	Dietary Fiber g
Grapefruit, 1/2 med.	154	5.5	50	I	14	0	0	6
Green beans, 3/4 cup cut	83	3	14	I	2	0	0	3
Green Onion, 1/4 cup chopped	25	I	7	0	I	0	0	0
Honeydew, 1/10 med.	134	5	50	I	12	0	50	I
Iceberg lettuce, 1/6 med. head	89	3	20	I	4	0	10	I
Kiwifruit, 2 med.	148	5.5	90	I	18	I	0	4
Leaf lettuce, 1 1/2 cups shredded	85	3	12	I	I	0	40	I
Lemon, I med.	58	2	18	0	4	0	10	0
Lime, I med.	67	2.5	20	0	7	0	I	3
Mushrooms, 5 med.	84	4	25	3	3	0	0	0
Nectarine, I med.	140	5	70	I	16	I	0	3
Onion, I med.	148	5.5	60	I	14	0	10	3
Orange, I med.	154	5.5	50	I	13	0	0	6
Peach, 2 med.	174	6	70	I	19	0	0	I
Pear, I med.	166	6	100	I	25	I	I	4
Pineapple, 2 slices, 3" diameter 3/4" thick	112	4	90	I	21	I	10	2
Plum, 2 med.	132	4.5	70	I	17	I	0	I
Potato, I med.	148	5.5	110	3	23	0	10	3
Radishes, 7	85	3	20	0	3	0	35	0
Strawberries, 8 med.	147	5.5	50	I	13	0	0	3
Summer squash, 1/2 med.	98	3.5	20	I	3	0	0	I
Sweet corn, kernels from I med. ear	90	3	75	3	17	I	15	I
Sweet potato, I med., 5" long, 2" diameter	130	4.5	140	2	32	0	15	3
Tangerine, 2 med., 2 3/8" diameter	168	6	70	I	19	0	2	2
Tomato, I med.	148	5.5	35	I	6	I	10	I
Watermelon, 1/18 med.; 2 cups diced	280	10	80	I	19	0	10	I

Source: U.S. Food and Drug Administration

NUTRITIONAL VALUE OF DAIRY PRODUCTS

	Serving Size	Calories	Protein g	Fat g	Cholesterol mg	Sodium mg	Calcium mg
MILK							
Skim milk	1 cup	89	8.0	0.4	5	128	303
Buttermilk	1 cup	92	8.1	2.4	10	212	293
1% milk	1 cup	102	8.0	2.7	10	122	300
2% milk	1 cup	122	8.1	4.7	20	122	298
Whole milk (3.25%)	1 cup	150	8.1	8.1	34	120	291
CREAM/EVAPORATED MILK							
Cream (heavy whipping)	1 tbsp.	52	0.3	5.6	20	6	10
Evaporated skim milk	1 oz.	23	2.3	tr.	1	35	87
Evaporated whole milk	½ cup	137	7.0	7.9	10	118	252
ICE CREAM							
Vanilla ice milk (soft serve)	½ cup	111	4.0	2.3	7.5	163	274
Vanilla ice cream (12% fat)	1 cup	278	5.3	16.4	80	53	164
BUTTER							
Sweet	1 tbsp.	107	0.9	12.2	39	1	3
Salted	1 tbsp.	108	0.1	12.2	33	124	4
YOGURT/SOUR CREAM/CREAM CHEESE							
Plain yogurt	1 cup	141	7.9	7.7	30	107	275
Low-fat plain yogurt (with nonfat milk solids)	1 cup	143	11.9	3.4	14	159	415
Low-fat flavored yogurt	1 cup	194	11.2	2.8	11	149	389
Low-fat fruited yogurt	1 cup	231	9.9	2.5	10	133	345
Sour cream, cultured	1 tbsp.	26	0.4	2.5	5	6	14
Cream cheese (2 tbsp.)	1 oz.	99	2.1	9.9	34	84	23

NUTRITIONAL VALUE OF DOMESTIC CHEESE

	Serving Size	Calories	Protein g	Fat g	Cholesterol mg	Sodium mg	Calcium mg
Cottage (1% fat)	1 cup	163	28.0	2.3	9	918	138
Cottage (2% fat)	1 cup	203	31.1	4.4	18	918	154
Cottage (4% fat)	1 cup	239	30.5	9.5	34	516	211
Ricotta (part skim)	½ cup	171	13.8	9.8	40	155	337
Ricotta (whole milk)	½ cup	216	14.5	16.1	63	104	257
Mozzarella (part skim)	1 oz.	72	6.9	4.5	16	132	183
Mozzarella (low moisture/ part skim)	1 oz.	78	7.7	4.8	15	148	205
Mozzarella (low moisture)	1 oz.	89	6.1	6.9	25	116	161
Mozzarella (whole milk)	1 oz.	79	5.4	6.1	22	104	145
Parmesan	1 oz.	111	10.1	7.3	19	454	336
Cheddar	1 oz.	112	7.0	9.1	30	197	211
Colby	1 oz.	110	6.7	9.0	27	169	192
Swiss	1 oz.	106	7.7	7.8	26	199	259
Provolone	1 oz.	98	7.4	7.3	19	245	212
Blue	1 oz.	103	6.0	8.5	21	390	88
Brie	1 oz.	94	5.8	7.8	28	176	52
Feta	1 oz.	74	4.0	6.0	25	312	138
Brick	1 oz.	103	6.2	8.5	25	157	204
Muenster	1 oz.	104	6.6	8.5	27	178	203
Monterey Jack	1 oz.	105	6.8	8.5	30	150	209
Fontina	1 oz.	109	7.2	8.7	32	—	154
Edam	1 oz.	87	7.7	5.7	25	270	225
Gouda	1 oz.	100	7.0	7.7	32	229	196
Cold pack	1 oz.	93	5.5	6.8	18	270	139
American, pasteurized processed	1 oz.	107	6.5	8.4	27	318	195

Source: Bowes & Church's Food Values of Portions Commonly Used
Compiled By: Wisconsin Milk Marketing Board with Wisconsin Dairy Council

NUTRITIONAL VALUE OF POULTRY
(per 3 oz. [100 g] edible, cooked, skinless)

	Calories g	Protein g	Carbo-hydrate g	Fat g	Saturated Fatty Acids g	Cholesterol mg	Sodium mg
CHICKEN							
Breast, baked	116	24	0	2	0	72	63
Drumstick, baked	132	23	0	3	1	79	81
Thigh, baked	150	21	0	7	2	81	75
Whole, roasted	135	23	0	4	1	76	73
Wing, baked	149	23	0	6	2	72	78
TURKEY							
Breast, baked	119	26	0	1	0	55	44
Drumstick, baked	143	24	0	4	1	67	80
Thigh, baked	142	23	0	5	2	66	71
Whole, roasted	129	25	0	3	1	64	59
Wing, baked	137	26	0	3	1	60	76

Serving Size: 3 oz. boneless, cooked, skinless portion roasted, baked, broiled/grilled, microwaved, stir fried, or cooked in liquid—without additional fat, salt, sodium, or sauces.
Source: USDA Handbook 8–5 and research conducted in cooperation with USDA.

Developed by the Food Marketing Institute, National Broiler Council, and National Turkey Federation in cooperation with the National Grocers Association and National-American Wholesale Grocers' Association, 1992.

NUTRITIONAL VALUE OF SEAFOOD
(per 3 oz. [100 g])

	Calories	Protein g	Fat g	Cholesterol mg	Sodium mg	Iron mg
SALTWATER FISH						
Anchovy (raw)	131	20.35	4.84	—	104	3.25
Bluefish	124	20.04	4.24	59	60	0.48
Blue runner (crevalle)	98	20.7	1.7	—	83	—
Butterfish	146	17.28	8.02	65	89	0.50
Bonito	111	20.5	2.5	37	—	12.15
Cod						
Atlantic cod	82	17.81	0.67	43	54	0.38
Pacific cod	82	17.90	0.63	37	71	0.26
Croaker	104	17.78	3.17	61	56	0.37
Crevalle jack	94	18.8	1.9	—	—	8.0
Cusk	87	18.99	0.69	41	31	0.83
Dolphin	85	18.50	0.70	73	88	1.13
Eel (mixed species)	184	18.44	11.66	126	51	0.50
Flounder (mixed species)	91	18.84	1.19	48	81	0.36
Golden kingklip	74	14.7	0.3	—	—	—
Greenland turbot	99	16.9	3.5	—	—	—
Grouper	92	19.38	1.02	37	53	0.89
Haddock	87	18.91	0.72	57	68	1.05
Halibut	110	20.81	2.29	32	54	—
Hawaiian fish						
Ahi (bigeye tuna)	108	23.38	0.95	45	37	0.73
Mahi mahi (Dolphin fish)	94	19.3	1.1	—	170	—
Oho (Hawaiian wahoo)	124	24.1	2.3	—	82	—
Opakapaka (pink snapper)	102	21.9	0.9	—	54	—
Herring						
Atlantic	158	17.96	9.04	60	90	1.10
Pacific	195	16.39	13.88	77	74	1.12
Ling	87	18.99	0.64	—	135	0.65
Lingcod	85	17.66	1.06	52	59	0.32
Mackerel						
Atlantic	205	18.60	13.89	70	90	1.63
King	105	20.28	2.00	53	158	1.78
Pacific jack	157	20.07	7.89	47	86	1.16
Spanish	139	19.29	6.30	76	59	0.44
Monkfish	76	14.48	1.52	25	18	0.32

	Calories	Protein g	Fat g	Cholesterol mg	Sodium mg	Iron mg
Mullet	117	19.35	3.79	49	65	1.02
Ocean catfish	103	17.60	3.60	—	100	—
Ocean perch						
Atlantic	94	18.62	1.63	42	75	0.92
Pacific	91	18.50	1.40	—	70	—
Orange roughy	126	14.70	7.00	20	63	0.18
Pollock						
Atlantic	92	19.44	0.98	71	86	0.46
Alaskan	81	17.18	0.80	71	94	0.23
Pompano	164	18.48	9.47	50	65	0.60
Porgy (scup)	105	18.88	2.73	—	42	0.53
Redfish	117	18.50	4.80	—	81	—
Rockfish (mixed)	94	18.75	1.57	35	60	0.41
Sablefish	195	13.41	15.30	49	56	1.28
Salmon (raw)						
Chinook	180	20.06	10.44	66	47	0.71
Coho	146	21.62	5.95	39	46	0.70
Pink	116	19.94	3.45	52	67	0.77
Sockeye	168	21.30	8.56	62	47	0.47
Sardines						
Atlantic canned in oil, drained	208	24.62	11.45	142	505	2.92
Pacific canned in tomato sauce, dr.	178	16.35	11.98	61	414	2.30
Sea bass (mixed)	97	18.43	2.00	41	68	0.29
Sea trout (mixed)	104	16.74	3.61	83	58	0.27
Shad	197	16.93	13.77	—	51	0.97
Shark (mixed species)	130	20.98	4.51	51	79	0.84
Skate (ray)	89	19.60	0.70	—	90	7.50
Snapper (mixed)	100	20.51	1.34	37	64	0.18
Sole (mixed)	91	18.84	1.19	48	81	0.36
Spot	123	18.51	4.90	—	29	0.32
Striped bass	97	17.73	2.33	80	69	0.84
Swordfish	121	19.80	4.01	39	90	0.81
Tilefish	96	17.50	2.31	—	53	0.25
Tuna						
Albacore	177	25.30	7.60	—	40	—
Bluefin	144	23.33	4.90	38	39	1.02
Skipjack	103	22.00	1.01	47	37	1.25
Yellowfin	108	23.38	0.95	45	37	0.73
Whitefish	134	19.09	5.86	60	51	0.37
Whiting (mixed)	90	18.31	1.31	67	72	0.34

	Calories	Protein g	Fat g	Cholesterol mg	Sodium mg	Iron mg
FRESHWATER FISH						
Burbot	90	19.31	0.81	60	97	0.90
Carp	127	17.83	5.6	66	49	1.24
Catfish (channel)	116	18.18	4.26	58	63	0.97
Lake trout	148	20.77	6.61	58	52	1.50
Lake whitefish	140	18.50	7.20	—	52	—
Pike						
Northern	88	19.26	0.69	39	39	0.55
Walleye	93	19.14	1.22	86	51	1.30
Rainbow trout	118	20.55	3.36	57	27	1.90
Shad	197	16.93	13.77	—	51	0.97
Smelt	97	17.63	2.42	70	60	0.90
Tilapia	98	18.50	2.40	—	52	—
SHELLFISH						
Abalone	105	17.10	0.76	85	301	3.19
Clams						
(raw, mixed						
species)	74	12.77	0.97	34	56	13.98
Crab (raw)						
Blue	87	18.06	1.08	78	293	0.74
Dungeness	86	17.41	0.97	59	295	0.37
King	84	18.29	0.60	42	836	0.59
Snow	90	18.50	1.18	55	539	—
Crayfish	89	18.66	1.06	139	53	2.45
Lobster						
Northern	90	18.80	0.90	95	—	—
Spiny	112	20.60	1.51	70	177	1.22
Mussels (blue)	86	11.90	2.24	28	286	3.95
Oysters						
Eastern & Gulf	69	7.06	2.47	55	112	6.70
Pacific	81	9.45	2.30	—	106	5.11
Scallops (mixed)	88	16.78	0.76	33	161	0.29
Shrimp (mixed)	106	20.31	1.73	152	148	2.41
Snails (unspec. raw)	75	14.40	1.90	—	—	25.00
Squid	92	15.58	1.38	233	44	0.68

Data from USDA Handbook Eight (1987) *Composition of Foods: Finfish and Shellfish Products* and from *Chemical and Nutritional Composition of Finfishes, Whales, Crustaceans, Mollusks, and Their Products,* Sidwell, NOAA Technical Memorandum NMFS F/SEC-11, U.S. Department of Commerce, 1981.

NUTRITIONAL VALUE OF MEATS—BEEF, VEAL, PORK, AND LAMB
(per 3 oz. [100 mg] edible, cooked, closely trimmed of fat)

	Calories	Protein g	Carbo-hydrate g	Fat g	Saturated Fatty Acids g	Cholesterol mg	Sodium mg
BEEF							
Brisket, point half, braised	222	24	0	13	5	77	65
Chuck, arm pot roast, braised	183	28	0	7	3	86	56
Chuck, blade roast, braised	213	26	0	11	4	90	60
Ground beef, regular (73%) broiled, med.	246	20	0	18	7	76	70
Ground beef, lean (83%) broiled, med.	217	22	0	14	5	71	59
Loin, sirloin steak, broiled	165	26	0	6	2	76	56
Loin, tenderloin steak, broiled	179	24	0	9	3	71	54
Loin, top, broiled	176	24	0	8	3	65	58
Rib, large end roast, roasted	201	23	0	11	4	69	62
Rib, small end steak, broiled	188	24	0	10	4	68	59
Round, eye, roasted	143	25	0	4	2	59	53
Round, bottom, braised	178	27	0	7	2	82	43
Round, tip roast, roasted	157	24	0	6	2	69	55
Round, top steak, broiled	153	27	0	4	1	71	52

	Calories	Protein g	Carbo-hydrate g	Fat g	Saturated Fatty Acids g	Cholesterol mg	Sodium mg
VEAL							
Cutlets, unbreaded, pan fried	156	28	0	4	1	91	65
Loin chop, roasted	149	22	0	6	2	90	82
Rib roast, roasted	151	22	0	6	2	97	82
Shoulder, arm steak, braised	171	30	0	5	1	132	76
Shoulder, blade steak, braised	168	28	0	6	2	135	86
PORK							
Loin, center chop, broiled	172	26	0	7	3	70	51
Loin, country style ribs, roasted	210	23	0	13	5	79	25
Loin, top chop, boneless, broiled	173	26	0	7	2	68	55
Loin, rib chop, broiled	186	26	0	8	3	69	55
Loin, sirloin roast, roasted	183	25	0	9	3	73	54
Loin, tenderloin, roasted	139	24	0	4	1	67	48
Loin, top roast, roasted	165	26	0	6	2	66	38
Shoulder, blade steak, broiled	193	23	0	11	4	80	63
Spareribs, braised	338	25	0	26	9	103	79
Ground pork, broiled	252	22	0	18	7	80	62

	Calories	Protein g	Carbo-hydrate g	Fat g	Saturated Fatty Acids g	Cholesterol mg	Sodium mg
LAMB							
Leg, whole, roasted	162	24	0	7	2	76	58
Loin, chop, broiled	183	25	0	8	3	80	71
Shank, fore, braised	159	26	0	5	2	89	63
Shoulder, arm chop, broiled	170	24	0	8	3	78	70
Shoulder, blade chop, broiled	179	22	0	10	3	78	75
Rib, roast, roasted	197	22	0	11	4	74	69

Serving Size: 3 oz.—well trimmed of fat—cooked portion roasted, baked, broiled/grilled, stir fried, or cooked in liquid without additional fat, salt, sodium or sauces.
Source: USDA Handbook 8-10 revised 1992 (pork) and USDA Handbook 8-17 revised 1989 (lamb).

Developed by the Food Marketing Institute, American Meat Institute, National Live Stock and Meat Board in cooperation with the National Grocers Association and National-American Wholesale Grocers Association, 1992.

NUTRITIONAL VALUE OF GAME MEATS
(per 3 oz. [100 g])

	Calories	Protein g	Total Fat g	Saturated Fatty Acids g	Cholesterol mg	Sodium mg
Antelope, cooked, roasted	127	25	2.27	.83	107	46
Bear, cooked, simmered	220	27.5	17.38	—	—	—
Buffalo, cooked, roasted	111	26	5.3	2.3	49	48
Boar, cooked, roasted	136	24	3.7	1.1	—	—
Caribou, cooked, roasted	142	25	3.8	1.4	93	51
Deer, cooked, roasted	134	26	2.7	1	95	46
Goat, cooked, roasted	122	23	2.6	.8	64	73
Moose, cooked, roasted	114	25	.8	.3	66	58
Rabbit (domesticated), cooked, roasted;	167	25	7	2	70	40
cooked, stewed	175	26	7	2.1	73	31
Rabbit (wild), cooked, stewed	147	28	3	.9	104	38
Squirrel, cooked, roasted	147	26	4	1	103	102
Duck, cooked and roasted flesh and skin, ½ duck	1,287	72	108	37	320	—
Pheasant, breast meat only, raw, ½ breast	243	44	6	2	—	—
Quail, breast meat only, raw, 1 breast	69	13	1.7	.5	—	—
Squab, breast meat only, raw, 1 breast	135	22	5	1.2	91	—

Source: USDA Handbook no. 8-17

▲▲▲

INDEX

250

Rice (*cont'd*)
  wehani and brown, with figs and scallions, 93–
    94
Risotto
  blushing pink, with Barolo wine, 161–62
  saffron-scented, with Portobello mushrooms,
    159–60
Ritz-Carlton hotels, 216–17
Roasted cod with peppers, onions, and new po-
    tatoes, 138–39
Romano, Michael, 220
Rosemary
  focaccia with onions, feta cheese, and, 86–
    87
  -juniper sauce, brochettes of venison with, 151–
    52
Royal Caribbean Cruise Line, 215

Safeway Stores, 192–93, 229
Saffron-scented risotto with Portobello mush-
    rooms, 159–60
Salad bars, 29–30, 198
Salad dressings, 117–18
  apricot vinaigrette, 125–26
  cilantro-lime, 123
  creamy tarragon, 127
  honey-Dijon, 124
  lemony dill, 122–23
  reduced-calorie or fat-free varieties, 201
  reducing fats in, 126
  sesame, 121–22, 124–25
Salads, 117–18
  chilled asparagus and grape, 118–19
  grilled Bangkok beef, 149–50
  Italian bread (*panzanella*), 119–20
  lamb, with green beans, 155–56
  lively two-tone potato, 113
  minty jalapeño rice, 94–95
  at salad bars, 29–30, 197–98
  sesame-dressed field greens with apples and wa-
    ter chestnuts, 121–22
  shocking pink rice, 95–96
  spinach, citrus, and goat cheese, 120–21
  warm barley-vegetable, 96–97
Salt, 23, 40–41
Saltwater fish, nutritional value of, 238–39. *See
    also* Fish
Sauces. *See also* Broths; Dips
  applesauce, Granny's, 129–30

blueberry, 130–31
fish (nam pla), 107, 149
rosemary-juniper, brochettes of venison with,
    151–52
Tamari or soy, 41
tomato, 127–29
Savory peppered corn muffins, 84–85
Scallions, wehani and brown rice with figs and,
    93–94
Scarlet runner beans, 100–101
Seafood. *See* Fish
Seasoned Italian tomatoes, 72
Seasonings. *See* Herbs and seasonings
Seeds
  poppy, lemon bundt cake with, 181–82
  poppy, yogurt-chive batter bread with, 83–
    84
  sesame, salad dressing with, 124–25
  squash, 14
Selection tips
  Bread, Cereal, Rice, and Pasta Group, 8–10
  Fats, Oils, and Sweets Group, 22–24
  frozen foods, 29, 194–97
  Fruit Group and Vegetable Group, 15, 29–30,
    198
  labels, 202
  Meat, Poultry, Fish, Dry Beans, Eggs, and Nuts
    Group, 20–22, 199
  menu literacy, 221
  Milk, Cheese, and Yogurt Group, 16–19, 198
  packaged foods, 200–202
  restaurant cuisine (*see* Restaurants)
  snacks, 29, 196
  supermarkets and Food Guide Pyramid pro-
    grams, 192–94
  Supermarket Savvy newsletter, 191–92
  time-saving, 29–30
Servings
  of fruits, 28, 34
  of grains, cereals, breads, and pasta, 34
  of meat, poultry, fish, dry beans, and protein
    alternatives, 36
  of milk, cheese, and yogurt, 35–36
  Pyramid Equivalents for, 41–43
  ranges of, 5, 6, 38
  sizes of, 32–38
  using fats, oils, and sweets sparingly, 37–38
  of vegetables, 28, 35
  visual cues to sizes of, 33